GLUTEN FREE FOR LIFE

Gluten Free for Life

Celiac Disease, Medical Recognition, and the Food Industry

Emily K. Abel

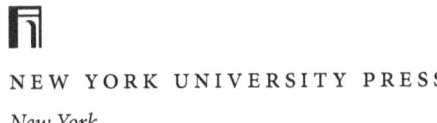

NEW YORK UNIVERSITY PRESS
New York

NEW YORK UNIVERSITY PRESS
New York
www.nyupress.org

© 2025 by New York University
All rights reserved

Please contact the Library of Congress for Cataloging-in-Publication data.
ISBN: 9781479834914 (hardback)
ISBN: 9781479834938 (paperback)
ISBN: 9781479834969 (library ebook)
ISBN: 9781479834952 (consumer ebook)

This book is printed on acid-free paper, and its binding materials are chosen for strength and durability. We strive to use environmentally responsible suppliers and materials to the greatest extent possible in publishing our books.

Manufactured in the United States of America

10 9 8 7 6 5 4 3 2 1

Also available as an ebook

CONTENTS

Introduction	1
1. The Rise and Fall of Celiac Disease in the United States	15
2. Gluten-Free Food: Trivial Fad or Medical Necessity?	31
3. Is It Really Gluten Free? Clarifying the Claims	52
4. Patient Advocacy, Corporate Funding, and the Cheerios Debacle	69
5. "You're Not Crazy": Getting—or Not Getting—a Diagnosis	93
6. Barriers to Adherence	113
7. Glutened!	125
8. "An Alien in a Strange World": Living and Working with Celiac Disease	143
Conclusion	167
Acknowledgments	175
Notes	177
Index	209
About the Author	219

Introduction

Celiac disease has touched my life in various ways. We now know that celiac is a serious, hereditary autoimmune disorder. Although the disease is considered gastrointestinal, it can affect many of the body's systems. As a result, the symptoms are extremely various, including anemia, bloating, brain fog, constipation, delayed growth in children, depression, diarrhea, fatigue, infertility, itchy skin, neuropathy, and vomiting. If left untreated, the disease may lead to certain kinds of cancers. The only remedy is lifelong avoidance of gluten, a protein found in wheat, rye, and barley. Celiac currently affects approximately 1 percent of the population, but evidence indicates that the incidence is increasing. Most people with the disease remain undiagnosed.[1]

That information was unavailable in 1947 when my younger sister, then three years old, was diagnosed with celiac. I am not sure whether my mother or our pediatrician reached that conclusion or on what basis either one did so. I do remember, however, that Peggy could not eat cake or corn on the cob, that bananas constituted a large part of her diet, and that her regimen did not seem unusual because some of my parents' friends' children had to abide by the same rules. I also remember looking forward to her fifth birthday because we had been told that she would be declared cured on that day. Years later, when I decided to attend public health school, my mother suggested that because I already had a history PhD, I should investigate why celiac seemed to have disappeared.

I wish I had followed her advice because I would have discovered that celiac disease is still with us and might not have assumed that my youngest daughter Heather's stomach aches were a normal part of childhood and her poor teeth just bad luck. When various other health problems arose in her twenties, I might have insisted more firmly that she consult a doctor. And in 2000, when she was thirty and called to tell me that she had just been diagnosed with celiac, I would not have assured her that she would outgrow it in a few years. I also would have followed her instructions more assiduously before she came home to visit and understood why the bread crumbs lying around infuriated her.

It was not easy to live with celiac in 2000. Almost no one Heather met had heard of the disease. The little available gluten-free food tasted like cardboard and could be found only in expensive health-food stores. No support groups or Internet sites provided practical information. The dietitian Heather consulted recommended a certain brand of gluten-free bread but had nothing else to offer.

Because there is a strong genetic predisposition to celiac disease, Heather's diagnosis also had ramifications for our entire family. We began to speculate that the same ailment had affected my mother. She had had bizarre eating habits throughout her life, often seemed to have gastrointestinal problems, and died from a kind of non-Hodgkin's lymphoma strongly linked to untreated celiac. If she did indeed have celiac, she probably would have experienced a raft of symptoms no doctor could explain. Then three of my siblings and some of their children realized that gluten upset their stomachs, too. (Ironically, Peggy was not among that group.) I was able to convince one niece who was living with me at the time that she had to consult a gastroenterologist and get tested. Most of my other relatives decided to avoid the arduous diagnostic process a doctor would prescribe, first a "gluten challenge" (eating a sizable amount of gluten for six weeks), followed by a blood test and, finally, if that was positive, an intestinal biopsy. They knew what they needed to do to feel better and doubted a doctor could help.

By contrast, my daughter Laura understood that she could not afford to be so lax when her daughter Emma began to complain of stomach aches at a young age. For several years, however, the pediatrician dismissed Laura's concerns, arguing that celiac was extremely rare, that stomach problems were common in childhood, and that Emma's difficulties undoubtedly stemmed from anxiety. Unaware of celiac's genetic component, the doctor ridiculed the notion that her aunt's diagnosis meant that Emma was at higher risk than other children. When Laura finally prevailed and the doctor referred Emma to a gastroenterologist, she underwent the prescribed diagnostic procedure, and we learned she had celiac. Not leaving anything to chance, Laura asked the gastroenterologist to order tests for herself and her son Max; they both were positive. I, too, was tested but discovered, to everyone's great surprise, that I did not have celiac.

By 2010, when Laura and her children received diagnoses, life with celiac had become somewhat easier. After a 2003 study demonstrated that the disease was far more prevalent than previously assumed, public and medical awareness grew. Gluten-free food had become more available and affordable. But as celebrities began to tout the benefits of eliminating gluten even for those without relevant medical conditions, the media circulated jokes about the diet. And rigorous adherence to a gluten-free diet remained exceedingly difficult. Because celiacs must avoid even the smallest crumb of gluten, many refuse to eat at friends' houses or restaurants or participate in potlucks.[2] Before 2014, no standards existed for the amount of gluten that could be contained in packaged food labeled "gluten free." The standards established by the Food and Drug Administration that year did not cover restaurants. Emma and Max were first children and then adolescents, anxious not to appear any different from their peers. A public-interest lawyer, Laura had a second full-time job, providing special food at home and ensuring her children's safety when they were away. This book explains why members of my family had such different experiences contending with the same diagnosis.

The Food Industry

A distinctive feature of celiac disease is that physicians have a marginal place in its management. Social historians of medicine argue that the rise of medical authority was intimately connected to the discovery of diagnostic technologies. In earlier centuries, patients' accounts figured prominently in clinical assessments. In the absence of virtually all diagnostic technologies, doctors had to listen to patients' narratives about their bodies. The second half of the nineteenth century, however, witnessed the introduction of stethoscopes and thermometers. By the 1920s, hospital doctors had access to the EKG, blood pressure cuff, and X-ray machines. And today, physicians can rely on technologies that produce even more precise information.[3] The 1952 discovery of a diagnostic tool for celiac disease was thus a major event, allowing doctors to discern distinct pathological changes rather than rely on patients' self-reports.

But diagnosis is especially powerful when it can lead to treatment and prognosis.[4] In the case of celiac disease, doctors can do neither. Because celiac is a lifelong condition, prognostication is irrelevant. The only remedy is a gluten-free diet, and adherence depends largely on individual and socioeconomic factors over which doctors have no control. Like many of my family members, some people diagnose themselves, trusting their own subjective, or embodied, knowledge and dispensing with medical certification and advice. Although the American Gastroenterological Association recommends that doctors regularly monitor patients after diagnosis, most people manage the disease on their own.[5] And even those who do consult doctors about celiac must remain vigilant, carefully scrutinizing all food labels and constantly surveilling their bodies to determine if they inadvertently have ingested gluten.

Unlike the medical profession, the food industry, a commercial enterprise, occupies a central place in the lives of people with celiac. Sociologist Eliot Freidson notes that one of the key elements of professionalism is "an ideology that asserts greater commitment to doing good work than to economic gain and the quality rather than the economic efficiency of work." Freidson acknowledges that this is an "intellectual construct and not a portrayal of any real occupation."[6] Indeed, numerous observers note that the line between medicine and commercialism recently has blurred. Rather than adhering strictly to the standards set by their peers, doctors increasingly view their patients as consumers and seek to satisfy their demands. No longer touting their superiority to business people, some even engage in advertising, a practice earlier generations of physicians deplored.[7] Nevertheless, the primary obligation of physicians is to their patients, not to shareholders.

The issue of overproduction highlights the contrast between the food industry and medicine. Fifty years ago, overeating replaced malnutrition as the major concern of food experts in affluent countries. The rising toll of the obesity epidemic has heightened that concern. Although obesity is responsible for various serious chronic diseases, most notably type 2 diabetes and coronary heart disease, the food industry has consistently encouraged Americans to eat larger portions and at more times of the day and resisted all attempts to urge us to eat less, especially of unhealthy products.[8] The Dietary Guidelines issued every five years by the Department of Agriculture and the Department of Health and Human Services illustrate the success of the industry's intense lobbying efforts. One reason most people find the guidelines so confusing is that groups representing food producers seek to obscure the message that highly processed food contributes to obesity.[9]

The closest analog in medicine is overtreatment. Doctors have called attention to the high level of unnecessary procedures for at least seven decades. In 1953 Paul Hawley, director of the American College of Surgeons, stated that "the public would be shocked if it knew the amount of unnecessary surgery performed." Urging Congress to hold a hearing on unnecessary surgery in 1976, the American Medical Association asserted that there were "2.4 million unnecessary operations performed on Americans at a cost of $3.9 billion and that 11,900 patients had died" as a result. Forty years later three surgeons wrote that "the existence of unnecessary surgery remains a daunting reality that continues to expose our patients to an unjustified surgical risk."[10] According to a 2019 study reported in *JAMA Network Open*, incidental findings on screening and diagnostic tests "may prompt cascades of testing and treatment that are of uncertain value."[11] Routine tests that have little or no value include

MRIs for uncomplicated back pain and prostate cancer screenings for men over age eighty.[12]

Physicians acknowledge that the profit motive partly explains unnecessary tests and procedures. Because doctors are reimbursed for every service, they earn more when they order more tests or provide more care. Those who own laboratories and outpatient surgical units have a direct financial incentive in providing unnecessary care. But there are other explanations as well, including patient requests, fear of liability, and difficulty accessing medical records.[13] Moreover, reports by physicians about unnecessary care typically conclude with recommendations for reform, such as educating both physicians and the public about the harms caused by overtreatment, identifying physician conflicts of interest, and discarding the fee-for-service reimbursement system.[14]

By contrast, it is extremely difficult to imagine major food corporations endorsing bans or restrictions on marketing campaigns that encourage consumers to consume more calories than they need. As Marion Nestle, a professor of food studies, nutrition, and public health, writes, "The primary mission of food companies, like that of tobacco companies, is to sell products. Food companies are not health or social service agencies, and nutrition becomes a factor in corporate thinking only when it can help sell food. The ethical choices involved in such thinking are considered all too rarely."[15] A critical feature of the celiac experience is that unless people have the time, skill, money, and inclination to prepare all their meals from basic ingredients, they must rely on an industry that has minimal interest in promoting their well-being.

The medical understanding of celiac changed dramatically between the 1940s and early 2000s, but a single theme dominates both periods—food-industry marketing played a major role in patients' experiences. In the 1940s, the United Fruit Company was able to exploit the pronouncements of the most prominent celiac doctor to sell bananas to the American public. Today, industry marketing overwhelms the nutritional advice physicians and dietitians deliver. Health professionals recommend that celiacs primarily eat simple foods that are naturally free of gluten. The websites of major celiac advocacy organizations, however, are filled with advertisements for ultraprocessed items. Those products also are promoted by the many celiac influencers on social media who earn money by forming partnerships with food companies.

People with celiac interact much less with the pharmaceutical industry than with food corporations, but drug makers are becoming increasingly important. Many advocacy organizations argue that because strict adherence to the celiac dietary regimen is extremely difficult, we should devote our efforts primarily to developing a drug treatment. But some groups exaggerate the promise of such a therapy. The drugs most likely to enter the market in the foreseeable future will serve as adjuncts to the gluten-free diet, not cure the disease.[16] My grandson tells me that he wishes he had an EpiPen for celiac. Just as people with food allergies can use an auto-injectable device to deliver epinephrine at the first sign of anaphylaxis, so he would like to have a pill to counter the serious and disagreeable effects of inadvertently consuming gluten. He understands, however, that he probably will have to avoid gluten as well as he can for the rest of his life.

A Disability Perspective

In addition to exploring the impact of the food and pharmaceutical industries on people with celiac, this book demonstrates that celiacs resemble those with other disabilities in various ways. Many are viewed—or view themselves—as burdensome. Declining invitations to social events that revolve around food, they often become socially marginalized. Historian Sarah F. Rose notes that "in many cultures, disability has been characterized as the inability to do productive labor, a charge that has limited the citizenship and social standing of people with disabilities."[17] Although labor and disability historians focus primarily on occupational illnesses and injuries, the primary concern of celiacs in the labor force is that their employment conditions will trigger or exacerbate symptoms.

Celiacs also share with other individuals with disabilities an inability to couch their experience in the form of a recovery narrative. That narrative wields such enormous power in our society that even people who deviate from its script must contend with it in some way.[18] Most people who scrupulously adhere to a gluten-free diet find that many symptoms fade or even disappear and that their small intestine eventually recovers. But celiac itself defies cure.

We can gain further insight into celiac by viewing it as one of the many disabilities (e.g., dyslexia, back aches, depression, and chronic fatigue) that lack externally observable symptoms. The absence of visible marks has some benefits, enabling people to camouflage problems they consider humiliating. Steven Lubet, a professor at the Northwestern Pritzker School of Law, asserted in 2015 that he was the only US law professor with chronic fatigue syndrome who had "gone public. I know there are other law professors, lawyers, and law students with the illness, because they have contacted me—always requesting anonymity for fear they will be belittled, ridiculed, or stigmatized."[19] Similarly, a recent study found that some people with celiac try to meet dates initially in places that do not serve food to avoid disclosing their condition.[20]

Disability scholars argue, however, that the disadvantages of invisibility far outweigh the advantages. Paula Kamen, a writer who lived with a headache for many years, commented that "whereas those with visible disabilities have long campaigned to 'fit in,' others who are regularly mistaken for 'normal' may long for a shared recognition of what they are going through."[21] A 1989 study found that 70 percent of people with facial pain reported that they sometimes wished that others could see how they felt.[22] Because people with celiac do not look sick, they cannot gain sympathy for the difficulties they confront. They also cannot easily distinguish themselves from the many individuals without medical diagnoses who choose gluten-free food. As a result, they often encounter derision when they request special meals. Fear of disclosure encourages some people with celiac to jeopardize their health by eating food containing gluten in public.[23] And concealment heightens the silence surrounding the disease. Because a central concern of advocates is to increase public and medical awareness of celiac, that is a major concern.

Looking Ahead

Chapter 1 demonstrates that, despite the widespread assumption that celiac has always been considered a rare disease in the United States, the condition captured widespread medical attention at the beginning of the twentieth century. The most famous celiac doctor was Sidney V. Haas, who recommended the consumption of large numbers of bananas, thereby promoting the marketing campaign of the United Fruit Company. In 1951, however, Dutch researchers reported that gluten caused celiac. Although European physicians quickly accepted that finding and continued to diagnose sizeable numbers of celiac cases, most US doctors lost interest in the disease.

The bulk of the book explores the years since the mid-1990s, when Italian gastroenterologists arriving in the United States helped to rekindle concern for celiac. Despite the many changes that have occurred in that period, rigorous, lifelong adherence to the gluten-free diet remains the only route to recovery. Chapters 2–4 examine the explosion of the gluten-free food market, the extent to which it has served the interests of the celiac community, and efforts by advocates to compel the food industry to reveal ingredients and clarify the meaning of the term "gluten free."

Chapter 2 argues that although the phenomenal growth of the gluten-free food industry has enormous implications for people with celiac, it did not arise from a concern with their needs and does not function for their benefit. Most products taste better than they did before, but they are expensive and unhealthy. Moreover, the enormous publicity surrounding the gluten-free diet has subjected all its adherents to derision.

People with celiac cannot make healthy food choices unless they have adequate information about the ingredients of the items they buy or consume. Chapter 3 examines the drive to improve product labeling. Although celiac advocates joined the campaign for passage of the 2004 Food Allergen Labeling and Consumer Protection Act, the food industry successfully prevented the inclusion of gluten in the act. Celiac advocates then turned their attention to pressing the Food and Drug Administration, first to establish standards for defining "gluten free" and then to enforce its ruling. That agency's failure to respond swiftly (if at all) to activist demands undermines the quality of life of people with celiac.

Like other health-advocacy organizations, those focusing on celiac seek to increase awareness of the disease, help sufferers manage the condition, and advocate for more research funding. After reviewing the accomplishments of the major celiac groups, chapter 4 asks to what extent the agendas of some have been distorted by funding from both the food and the pharmaceutical industries. The chapter also uses the example of Cheerios cereal produced by General Mills (GM) to illustrate how a company could continue to sow confusion after regulations defining "gluten free" were issued. Although celiac advocates have been united in the campaign for food labeling, they responded in different ways to GM's tactics.

Chapters 5–8 focus more directly on the difficulties celiacs experience attempting to adhere to the gluten-free diet. I use the word "adherence" rather than "compliance" to follow the recommendations of a growing number of researchers. The World Health Organization defines "adherence" as "the extent to which a person's behavior—taking medication, following a diet, and/or executing lifestyle changes—corresponds with the agreed recommendations from a healthcare provider." Unlike compliance, which implies that an individual passively follows medical advice, adherence "requires the patient's agreement to the recommendations."[24]

Chapter 5 demonstrates that because public and medical recognition of celiac has been slow, the condition remains greatly underdiagnosed. As a result, many people never learn that they must adhere to the gluten-free diet. Others wait for years to learn the name of their disease and the dangers gluten presents for them. The failure of physicians to offer dietary advice to newly diagnosed celiacs leaves many uncertain about how to proceed.

Chapter 6 argues that the many studies of adherence that focus on individual factors ignore the lived reality of certain groups. Adherence is virtually impossible for those who speak little or no English, are poor, live in food deserts, or reside in long-term institutions (most notably nursing homes and prisons).

Chapter 7 juxtaposes the accounts of social media influencers with those of other people with celiac to demonstrate why adherence does not always result in recovery. Although many celiacs report that they gradually begin to feel better after adopting a gluten-free diet, they live with the constant threat of inadvertently ingesting enough gluten to precipitate symptoms and damage the small intestine. The chapter explores the reasons why many celiacs hold themselves accountable for any gluten exposure despite inaccurate or misleading package labeling and unsafe restaurant practices.

Chapter 8 shows that strict adherence to the celiac dietary regimen can have severe repercussions for social and labor-force participation. Because social lives commonly revolve around food, many celiacs complain that their attempt to eliminate gluten results in loneliness and isolation. Although most celiacs can remain in the labor force, some jobs undermine workers' ability to follow dietary guidelines.

The conclusion uses the various meanings of the word "access" to summarize the book's basic themes.

Sources

This book relies on close analysis of numerous sources of data, including articles in both medical journals and the popular press, sociological, historical, and anthropological studies, the websites of major celiac organizations, policy reports, and patient narratives. My selection of those sources was informed by various disciplines, including food studies, disability studies, public health, and the medical humanities. To understand the perspective of people with celiac, I draw heavily on celiac.com, one of the first websites dedicated to that disease. Although celiac.com has grown significantly since its establishment in 1995, it has received harsh criticism from those who complain that its articles contain misleading information and its advertisements promote products that are unsafe for celiacs.[25] Nevertheless, its patient forums provide windows on the experiences of people with celiac. I use the forum "Coping with Celiac Disease," which calls itself a place where participants "share stories, techniques, and information to help others deal with the disease and the gluten-free diet." By January 1, 2023, the forum had received more than 150,000 posts. Both the screen names and personal information in the posts suggest that women are greatly overrepresented, as they are in other support groups. Given the nature of the sample, quantification is not appropriate. To protect confidentiality, I use pseudonyms rather than the screen names participants provided. The dates following quotations from the forum indicate when they were posted.

Because people are most likely to discuss their experiences, solicit information, and ask questions when they are dissatisfied, the forum may exaggerate the negative aspects of life with celiac. But the forum participants also represent a very privileged group of celiacs. Although some complain about inadequate access to health care and the cost of gluten-free products, none, as far as I can tell, is food insecure, incarcerated, or a nursing home resident. The level of writing in the posts indicates that the participants are fluent in English and have received enough education to understand nutritional advice and read food labels.

The comments I quote were posted between January 2005 and January 2022. Because celiac awareness spread (albeit slowly and haltingly) in the medical community in that seventeen-year period, I had expected that later participants would suggest that members of their social networks knew more about the disease than earlier participants did. Nevertheless, at the end of that period, as in the beginning, writers complained about the widespread misunderstanding of the severity of celiac and the extreme measures all sufferers must take to protect their health. I gained some insight into that issue when I first discussed this project with members of my history writing group. In the more than twenty years we had been meeting, I had mentioned celiac and its effect on my family at various times. But the members were stunned to learn that because even the smallest crumb of gluten can trigger symptoms and cause serious harm, adherence to the prescribed diet can affect every aspect of life. Moreover, gluten can lurk even in skin products and medications. A major goal of this book is to increase awareness of both the experiences of people with celiac and the reforms needed to keep them safe.

1

The Rise and Fall of Celiac Disease in the United States

Although the name "celiac disease" has been in existence since the late 1880s, the medical understanding of the disorder has changed dramatically since that time. The few brief histories of the disease begin with an 1888 paper entitled "On the Coeliac Affection," by the English doctor Samuel Gee. "There is a kind of chronic indigestion," he wrote, "which is met with in persons of all ages, yet is especially apt to affect children between one and five years old.... Signs of the disease are yielded by the faeces; being loose, not formed, but not watery; bulkier than the food taken would seem to account for." Some writers emphasize the prescience of Gee's comment: "If the patient can be cured at all, it must be by means of diet." But Gee's dietary recommendations have not stood the test of time. He fed one child "the best Dutch mussels daily." And he concluded that patients should be given "bread cut thin and well toasted on both sides."[1]

US Pioneers

In the late nineteenth and early twentieth centuries, physicians gained social legitimacy by allying themselves with an accumulation of dramatic bacteriological breakthroughs. As the status of all physicians increased, elite doctors (defined by both their own class background and that of their patients) tried to distance themselves from the rest by organizing themselves into specialties.[2] Lacking a particular body part over which to claim jurisdiction, pediatricians asserted authority over child welfare and development, during a period of unprecedented concern with both. The first child specialists organized the AMA Section on the Diseases of Children in 1880 and eight years later founded the independent American Pediatric Society. The establishment of pediatric journals and the growth in the size and number of hospitals specifically for babies and children also marked the emergence of the field.[3]

Luther Emmett Holt occupied a preeminent position among the second generation of pediatricians. His major hospital appointment was at Babies' Hospital of the City of New York (a charity facility that was later part of Columbia-Presbyterian Medical Center), where he served as medical director for several decades. His extensive publications list includes his widely used 1897 textbook, *Diseases of Infancy and Childhood*, and his extremely popular advice manual for mothers and nurses, which was translated into seventy-five languages.[4]

Holt also figured prominently in the development of the Rockefeller Institute for Medical Research. As the pediatrician of several Rockefeller children and a member of the same Fifth Avenue church as John D. Rockefeller Jr., Holt was uniquely poised to convince both him and his father of the need to establish a facility emulating and rivaling the institutes already existing in France, Germany, and England. With well-funded and fully equipped laboratories, those institutes had established European supremacy in scientific medicine. A similar project could bring equal glory to the US medical enterprise. Holt presented his proposal to John D. Rockefeller Jr. first on a long train trip they happened to take together and then at a dinner Holt organized at his home. Soon afterwards, he received a letter from Rockefeller containing a check from his father to inaugurate the institute. Its incorporation occurred in Holt's office in 1901, after which he served on the Board of Scientific Directors.

Although many people complain about doctors' lack of interest in nutrition today, the subject dominated Holt's concerns throughout his career. As he proclaimed in 1897, "Nutrition in its broadest sense is the most important branch of pediatrics. In no other field and at no other time in life does prophylaxis give such results as in the conditions of nutrition in infancy."[5] In his private practice, he dispensed detailed advice to mothers about infant feeding. Explaining his therapeutic regime at Babies' Hospital, he wrote, "To the matter of diet the closest attention is given, not only the exact nature and preparation of the food, but the precise dose and frequency of administration. The prescriptions for food are made with as much care and exactness as those for drugs."[6] The preoccupation with infant mortality at the time justified that conclusion. By the turn of the twentieth century, most doctors realized that death in the first months and years of life was not inevitable and that public health efforts could help to reduce the rate.[7] At Babies' Hospital, as at every other facility for infants, the major cause of mortality was gastrointestinal disease.[8]

Holt applied the name "chronic intestinal indigestion" to a particular set of symptoms. His interest in them can be explained in various ways. First, they included a distinctive type of diarrhea. One historian writes that doctors often described babies' bowel movements in exquisite detail, noting the "tiniest nuances in symptoms—color and texture of stools, severity of abdominal pain, amount of flatulence, and the presence or absence of vomiting, for example."[9] The stools of chronic intestinal indigestion were unusually soft and foul smelling.

Second, unlike other diarrheal diseases, this one seemed to be far more common among Holt's private patients than among the children he saw at the hospital.[10] Holt played a leading role in efforts to shift the focus of the movement to reduce infant mortality from broad environmental reform to maternal instruction.[11] Here was a disease, however, that seemed to strike the very children whose mothers were most likely to receive and follow his advice.

Finally, the disease may have both fascinated and disturbed Holt because the survivors invariably lagged far behind their age mates in physical development. Holt was one of the first physicians to argue that weight gain served as an accurate measure of nutritional status. His advice manual urged mothers to weigh babies every week, and his textbook provided guidelines physicians could use to gauge whether the growth was adequate.[12] Babies who failed to adhere to the standard and occasionally lost rather than gained pounds were thus a source of grave concern.

Although Holt never investigated the condition on his own, he encouraged three other physicians to do so. All three eventually played pivotal roles in the early history of what became known as celiac disease. The first was Christian Herter, whose 1908 book *On Infantilism from Chronic Intestinal Infection* described a condition "so clearly definable that few pediatricians with a practice among children will fail to recognize a few instances of this unmistakable and extreme manifestation of a morbid nutritional process." The most significant features of that condition included "an arrest in the development of the body," "the maintenance of mental powers and fair development of the brain," "marked abdominal distension," a "moderate grade of anaemia," the "rapid onset of physical and mental fatigue," and "various obtrusive irregularities referable to the intestinal tract," including extremely frequent and fatty stools.[13] Herter was not aware of the 1888 paper by Samuel Gee, and his name never appears in Herter's monograph. After its publication, however, communication between European and US researchers increased. Among the various labels attached to this condition in the early twentieth century was "Gee-Herter Disease."[14]

Herter anticipated that he would continue to pursue research on the disorder after the completion of his study. One avenue would be through a hospital connected to the Rockefeller Institute for Medical Research. Along with Simon Flexner, a professor of pathology at the University of Pennsylvania, Herter frequently pushed the other members of the Board of Scientific Directors to establish such a facility. But in 1902 he had begun to show disturbing symptoms, and by 1908 he was seriously ill. He died at the age of forty-five on December 15, 1908, two months after the official opening of the hospital. Nevertheless, the new hospital continued to feel his imprint. Following the plan he and Flexner had outlined, the hospital concentrated on five conditions. Four were diseases that captured widespread medical and popular attention: poliomyelitis, lobar pneumonia, syphilis, and heart disease. The fifth, included at Herter's behest, was intestinal infantilism. Among the first patients admitted to the hospital were several suffering from that disorder.[15] It is tempting to imagine the prominence intestinal infantilism might have been accorded had Herter survived. In the event, however, the disease soon faded from the hospital's agenda.

The two other physicians Holt encouraged to study this disease initially served as his assistants. In 1921 John Howland gave a presidential address to the American Pediatric Society entitled "Prolonged Intolerance to Carbohydrates." He began by noting that he chose the topic for three reasons, the "frequency of the condition," its "importance from the nutritional standpoint," and his desire "to stimulate an interest to inquire more deeply into a subject on which our present knowledge is disappointingly scanty." After discussing two types of carbohydrate intolerance, he focused on a third that was "perhaps the most striking and certainly the most persistent." That condition had a variety of explanations and names (including "chronic intestinal indigestion" and "intestinal infantilism"), but "the clinical picture" was "sufficiently characteristic." Howland's description closely mirrored that of Herter. A "child of 18 months or older" has "loose stools from time to time with loss of weight." The "relapses" become "increasingly severe," eventually resulting in "a condition of marked malnutrition." "Growth suffers," and the child remains "greatly below the average height."[16]

Howland's major contribution was to propose a new treatment. From "clinical experience," he had found that "of all the elements of the food carbohydrates is the one which must be excluded rigorously."[17] The diet he recommended had three stages. During the first, typically lasting a few days or weeks, children received only protein milk. The second stage was the longest. The "duration," Howland noted, could be "many months" or even "years." Now the protein milk was supplemented with other forms of protein, including "curd without whey, scraped meat, certain forms of cheese, egg white and eventually the whole egg." Although this diet was hardly "ideal," it was "adequate."[18]

The third stage, involving the introduction of carbohydrates, was the most difficult. One physician later recalled that "all . . . trembled in fear of the result."[19] Howland thus added carbohydrates "very gradually with the most careful observation of the digestive capacity." He acknowledged that the treatment was "time consuming," but the "patients well repay the effort expended on them. They do not remain semi-invalids. Many become vigorous and strong."[20]

Bananas

The third person Holt urged to investigate this intestinal disorder helped to associate it not with elite medical institutions but rather with the marketing efforts of a major food company. Three years after Howland's pediatric society address, Sidney V. Haas published an article in the *American Journal of Diseases of Children* titled "The Value of the Banana in the Treatment of Celiac Disease."[21] Reflecting the widespread belief that bananas were harmful for children, Holt had included them in his 1897 list of "forbidden" foods.[22] But public perceptions of the fruit had undergone a transformation since then. After its incorporation in 1899, the United Fruit Company (UFC) had quickly secured a dominant place in the burgeoning food industry by taking advantage of US imperialist ventures in the Caribbean and Latin America and technological innovations in pest control, transportation, and distribution. As the number of bananas arriving in US ports rapidly increased, the company launched a massive advertising campaign to transform the fruit's image. Once a rare luxury item, the banana gradually became an essential component of a healthy daily diet, even for children.[23]

The promotional drive relied heavily on medical endorsements. In 1917, the UFC published *The Food Value of the Banana*, a compilation of writings by doctors, public health officials, and nutritionists, testifying to the unique advantages of its product.[24] "It is well to bear in mind," declared Drs. Victor C. Myers and Anton R. Rose, that the banana's "caloric value is very high—in fact higher than that of any other common fruit in its natural state."[25] The *Journal of the American Medical Association* added that "this fruit is sealed by nature in practically germ-free and germ-proof packages," a major concern at a time of heightened alarm about the disease-bearing microbes circulating in the air.[26] Bananas also had universal appeal. "Children cry for them," proclaimed Dr. Frank Crane. "Negroes, Chinamen, college girls, octogenarians, invalids, brides and grooms, messenger boys, railroad presidents, bankers, janitors, prize fighters, and pacifists like them."[27] And they had unique therapeutic powers. A Kentucky physician had served bananas to typhoid fever patients "with the happiest results."[28] Drs. Myers and Rose found them "a particularly valuable food to employ in the dietetic treatment of nephritic patients with nitrogen retention."[29] Dr. W. Gilman Thompson, an "eminent authority on dietetics," successfully fed the fruit to "some fifty patients in the New York and Presbyterian Hospitals."[30]

Haas stated that he found particular inspiration in a 1917 article by Drs. Marshall C. Pease and Anton R. Rose refuting any lingering fears about the banana's dangers for children and investigating "the best ways of using it to get full nutritive value without digestive disturbances."[31] In his 1924 paper, Haas noted that he had first employed a banana treatment for a three-year-old girl with "a severe case of anorexia nervosa." Although she refused "all food," she "finally accepted a banana, with the result that other food was taken in a more or less normal amount within forty-eight hours."[32] Encouraged by that success, Haas turned his attention to the condition Holt had urged him to examine many years earlier. The term he used was a US adaptation of Samuel Gee's "coeliac."

Like Howland, Haas argued that children suffering from celiac disease must avoid all carbohydrates besides those in milk products. But he made "one exception, that is, sucrose, as it occurs in the extremely ripe banana." That fruit was "not only well tolerated, but rapidly changes the entire picture of the disease to one of well being."[33] Haas restricted the diet of his celiac patients to protein milk, broths, gelatin, meat, and, above all, bananas. Most children he treated consumed between four and eight bananas a day. In one case a two-year-old boy "took sixteen bananas daily, a short time after they had been prescribed."[34]

Although Haas first presented his findings at a meeting at the New York Academy of Medicine and then published them in a prestigious medical journal, his report bore a remarkable similarity to a popular line of health writing. Historian Harvey Levenstein notes that "the decades that straddled the turn of the [twentieth] century constituted a veritable Golden Age of food faddism." The recommended dietary change varied enormously, but advocates "usually shared a common characteristic: they bore personal witness to its efficacy. Almost invariably, proponents would tell of their own devastating health problems, miraculously cured by the proposed diet—mysterious or common physical or psychological ailments that had defied the greatest of modern medical minds had disappeared once certain foods were added or deleted from the diet." Food faddism, of course, had long existed, but the new knowledge about the chemical properties of foods allowed advocates to claim that their diets had undergone "impersonal scientific testing."[35]

Haas drew on clinical observations rather than personal experience, but he described the efficacy of bananas in the same exaggerated terms. "The difficulty in treating [celiac] cases is proverbial," he wrote, "relapses even after marked temporary progress being the regular experience." Because children with celiac could not absorb essential nutrients, the disease had a high case fatality rate. Haas, however, cured eight of the ten children he treated. The only two who died had been allowed to eat the wrong food.[36] The exactness of his advice endowed it with authority. He specified the precise amount of each food item and the hour at which it should be offered. Before-and-after photographs of Haas's most striking successes, excerpts from his case reports, charts demonstrating the steady increases in height and weight, and precise information about the nutritional properties of the prescribed diet also lent a scientific aura to his claims.[37]

Several of Haas's colleagues quickly embraced his advice. A 1928 article in the *American Journal of Nursing* noted that "the banana is being used by many pediatricians in the treatment of celiac disease." Because "the number of bananas given daily may become tiresome to a child," the author suggested that nurses "add the psychological touch" by providing historical "facts," which could be "sent on request from the United Fruit Company."[38]

Haas continued to investigate the medical benefits of bananas. Given the pediatric preoccupation with infant feeding at the time, it is perhaps unsurprising that he examined the fruit's role in bottle formulas. A 1931 article noted that he had used "banana powder . . . experimentally for over two years in several hundred cases" with excellent results. Compared with controls, infants fed with mixtures containing the powder have shown "an acceleration of the rate of growth in length." Haas postulated that the fruit's benefit lay in the special enzyme it contained, "capable of hydrolyzing" starch and "of converting cane sugar to invert sugar."[39]

Celiac disease remained his primary interest. By 1932, he had treated seventy-five sufferers. Those who followed his regime attained "full stature" and were eventually "capable of using a normal diet." Relapses were almost "always due to the introduction of some carbohydrate other than that of the banana."[40] Although he failed to indicate what proportion of the patients in his study had recovered, the *New York Times* proclaimed his treatment "an example of the rapidly developing science of finding in two or three commonplace articles of food a . . . natural 'medicine.'"[41]

But applause was not universal. John Lovett Morse, an emeritus Harvard Medical School professor, wrote in 1932 that since Haas first announced his treatment for celiac, "the articles on this subject in American medical literature have read like advertisements of the United Fruit Company." Morse's own analysis suggested that bananas lacked any special curative powers. Although the fruit represented "a fairly safe and convenient method of giving carbohydrates," there was "no reason" to believe it had "any specific action in the treatment of this condition."[42]

Morse may have found medical writing about celiac disease uncomfortably similar to UFC propaganda because that company quickly exploited Haas's study. The 1926 edition of *The Food Value of the Banana* included a lengthy summary of the report Haas had published two years earlier. In 1936, the company issued a new digest of scientific literature "with the object of enabling the busy physician, as well as the nutritionist and dietitian, to become quickly yet thoroughly acquainted with the published facts regarding the nutritive and therapeutic values of the banana."[43] All three of Haas's publications received prominent attention.[44]

After the outbreak of World War II, various forces combined to reduce the availability of bananas, including fears of German submarine attacks in the Caribbean, the conversion of fruit ships into military carriers, and the growing congestion of the national railway system. As the number of bananas in grocery stores plummeted, mothers of children with celiac disease panicked.[45] The *New York Times* reported on July 31, 1942, "Brooklyn police found twenty four ripe bananas in the borough yesterday after a frantic search for the fruit which was urgently needed for the diet of a 15-month-old baby suffering from celiac." The bananas were "delivered to Mrs. Rebecca Gottlieb" for "her infant daughter, Helena Roberta." The previous day, Mrs. Gottlieb had "walked the streets of her neighborhood for two and a half hours in vain while the borough police canvassed markets and stores in radio cars and on foot, before enlisting the aid of Nat Smillen, one of the borough's fruit and vegetable merchants." Smillen "suggested that the Brooklyn Terminal Market at Remsen and Foster Avenues, Brooklyn, be tapped. Here eight bananas were found." Smillen had even better luck himself. Searching his own warehouses, he discovered "'a treasure trove'—sixteen bananas."[46] Ten days later, *Newsweek* reported that the Canadian Colonial Airways had flown a bunch of bananas from New York to Montreal for "22-month-old Margo Bradley" and that Mrs. Valentine Dreschel had appealed to the *New York Journal-American* for help for her twenty-one-month-old son, John, "saying the baby's life depended upon his obtaining more bananas."[47]

Such stories presented a golden propaganda opportunity for the United Fruit Company, and it rapidly took advantage of them. A few days after the *Times* chronicled Mrs. Gottlieb's saga, the paper published a letter from Sidney V. Haas reassuring parents of celiac children that the UFC "is doing all that is possible to meet the situation" and urging them to contact the company for help.[48] A 1945 United Fruit Company ad featured a picture of one-year-old Ottile M. Schmelzer of Ozone Park, New

York, surrounded by bunches of bananas. "War or no war," the title read, "celiac babies get bananas." The accompanying text noted that "at the request of the United Fruit Company, the banana jobbers of the country set aside a portion of their scant supplies to take care of the needs of celiacs and others for whom doctors prescribe bananas."[49]

After the war ended, the UFC unleashed a new promotional campaign based on the cartoon character, Miss Chiquita Banana.[50] But medical themes continued to dominate the ads targeting at least some audiences. One placed in the *American Journal of Nursing* asked, "Doctor, would it be helpful to you in your practice to know that there is a food available at reasonable prices in the stores the year round having these attributes?" The answer, of course, was "bananas," and one of their many "attributes" was usefulness "in the dietary management of celiac disease."[51]

In 1949, the New York Academy of Medicine held a "Golden Jubilee World Tribute" honoring Haas's "fiftieth year of medical practice." Robert Moses, park commissioner of New York City, served as toastmaster. Speeches by leading pediatricians lauded Haas's major scientific achievements, most notably his "pioneering contribution to celiac therapy." The commemorative booklet published soon after the event declared Haas's discovery "so pivotal that it altered the prognosis of celiac" and "greatly aided physicians everywhere in treating the disease."[52]

The following year Haas published a new paper on celiac disease, this time with his physician-son Merrill. They noted that the contours of the disease had changed significantly since Sidney Haas had last published an article on the subject, in 1932. The 1938 identification of cystic fibrosis as a distinct clinical entity had removed some very sick children from the celiac label. But doctors also realized that the disorder could take relatively mild forms. The cases in Sidney Haas's original study all had extreme emaciation and distended abdomens. Those were now understood to be symptoms only of advanced disease. The description of the therapeutic power of bananas also was very different. Gone was any mention of a special enzyme capable of altering the type of sugar. The banana's "particular value in celiac disease" lay in "the fact that it is 20 percent carbohydrate and thus replaces better than any other fruit the excluded carbohydrates such as cereal, sugars, and potatoes." But the dietary regime remained largely unaltered, and its results continued to impress. Of the 370 cases the doctors had followed "over a period of some length," 270 (73 percent) were cured. An additional eighty-nine (24 percent) were "still being treated" and were "on the road to cure." Only eight (2.2 percent) failed to recover, and three (0.8 percent) died. Haas and his son were so certain of the merits of their therapy that they proposed a new definition of celiac disease: successful recovery of patients following the adoption of the banana diet.[53]

Then, in 1951, a year after the publication of that article, Dutch researchers reported their discovery that gluten caused celiac disease and the only effective treatment was a gluten-free diet.[54] Because patients could now safely eat all carbohydrates that did not contain the offending ingredient, bananas no longer had any special therapeutic role. Although European and Australian researchers quickly accepted the Dutch finding, many Americans remained skeptical. Haas was especially resistant. In 1963 he still asserted that his dietary regimen had "practically solved the problem of the successful treatment of celiac disease." True, the Dutch report had been "hailed as a demonstration of the etiologic factor of celiac disease," but "time has shown that it is only one of the causes of the celiac syndrome." Haas highlighted a recent study that found that nearly half of patients on a gluten-free diet "relapsed when gluten was used again." In addition, there were "reports of failures, crises, and occasional deaths." His therapy alone was able to achieve a "cure which is permanent without relapse."[55]

Technology

By the time Haas made those remarks, technological advances had confirmed the Dutch discovery. In 1956, Margot Shiner, a British-German physician, devised an intestinal biopsy capsule that could be used on children. Although the first capsules perforated the intestines of some very small infants, subsequent refinements gradually improved the procedure.[56] Various biopsy studies revealed that gluten was responsible for changes observed in the intestinal mucosa of children with celiac disease and that a gluten-free diet could reverse those changes. Researchers also were able to define celiac disease with greater precision than ever before. In 1962, L. Emmett Holt Jr. (a pediatrician who carried on the tradition of his more famous father) noted that the label previously had been attached to a "heterogeneous group of patients." He stressed in particular the need to eliminate all mild cases of chronic or recurrent diarrhea from the celiac definition.[57] We recall that, in 1950, Sidney Haas and his son noted that doctors recently had added those cases to the term.

Because physicians now had a diagnostic tool, they could rely on the discernment of distinct pathological changes rather than on clinical observation or patient (and parental) reports. One might therefore have expected the disease to gain new recognition and respect. European and Australian physicians continued to diagnose sizeable numbers of celiac cases. In the United States, however, the disease gradually faded from view. "Where Have All the Celiacs Gone?" asked gastroenterologist John D. Lloyd-Still in 1970. "The incidence" of the disease was "1 in 890 in Switzerland." A physician at the Melbourne Children's Hospital in Australia "reported seeing 90 new patients with celiac disease in a four-year interval." But the disease was "now a rare diagnosis in the United States." Lloyd-Still found only "three new celiac cases per year" at the Children's Memorial Hospital in Chicago "despite performing intestinal biopsies in all suspected cases."[58]

The contrast between the United States and other countries is especially striking in the area of research. Despite the widespread attention accorded the studies of Herter, Howland, and Haas, Americans had never dominated celiac disease study. But after the mid-1960s, the US role became especially marginal. Although US researchers made major discoveries, a 1996 study reported that Americans were authors of only 48 (less than 1 percent) of the 6,278 articles on celiac disease published between 1966 and 1995.[59] The disorder also vanished from the popular media. Searches in article databases revealed no mention of the disease in either popular magazines between 1969 and 1982 or the *New York Times* between 1964 (when Sidney V. Haas's obituary appeared) and 1980 (when Jane Brody briefly referred to celiac in her weekly health column).[60] And, of course, once a gluten-free diet supplanted Haas's banana regimen, the United Fruit Company lost all interest in the disorder. The ads that once had helped to publicize celiac disease now concentrated entirely on other issues.

Resurgence

Two Italian gastroenterologists who arrived in the United States in the mid-1990s helped to rekindle interest in celiac disease. Stefano Guandalini graduated from the University of Messina, Italy, in 1971 and worked in Italy for many years before moving to the University of Chicago Medical School in 1996. What he found stunned him: "Nobody really was ready to accept the 1 percent prevalence of celiac disease." He added that a prominent medical textbook reported that celiac affected only one in ten thousand people in the United States and that the disease was "mostly a European condition."[61] Seeking to alter that situation, Guandalini founded the University of Chicago Celiac Disease Center, which he directed for many years.

Alessio Fasano graduated from the University of Naples, Italy, in 1981 and moved to the University of Maryland Medical School in 1993. In 1999 he established the University of Maryland Center for Celiac Research.[62] That year he also published a major paper titled "Where Have All the American Celiacs Gone?," echoing the question posed by Lloyd-Still twenty-six years earlier. Using new serological tests, European researchers had discovered that celiac symptoms were far more varied than previously understood, that asymptomatic and silent forms of the disease exist, and that the disorder affects adults as well as children. As a result, epidemiological studies had demonstrated that the disease was prevalent throughout Europe. American researchers, however, continued to insist that the condition was rare in the United States.[63]

By 2003, Fasano was ready to answer his own question. Millions of Americans suffered from celiac disease, but the vast majority remained undiagnosed. He and his colleagues from several US medical centers concluded, "Celiac disease appears to be a more common but neglected disorder than has generally been recognized in the United States." The prevalence was 1:133, roughly comparable to that found in European countries.[64] Andrea Levario, a lawyer who was a major celiac advocate at the time, commented that the study "opened the doors for people paying much more attention" to celiac disease.[65] According to Google Scholar, the article has been cited nearly twenty-five hundred times.

In 2004, the year after Fasano's article appeared, celiac finally received US medical certification. The National Institutes of Health held a two-day Health Consensus Development Conference to present the "state of knowledge" about the disease. Celiac was now a very different disorder from the one that Herter and Haas had identified. An autoimmune disease affecting the gastrointestinal tract, celiac could lead to various serious problems if left untreated. The gold standard for diagnosis was a blood test followed by an endoscopy. The primary treatment was the exclusion of gluten from the diet. Although considered a childhood disease, it often presented in adulthood with a wide variety of symptoms. "Heightened awareness," especially among physicians and dietitians, was "imperative."[66] A survey published the following year explained why. Just 32 percent of physicians knew that the onset of celiac could occur in adulthood; although 90 percent knew that diarrhea was a common celiac symptom, most could not name other symptoms.[67]

Much has changed in the years since Fasano demonstrated that celiac was as widespread in the United States as in Europe. Twenty-one US hospitals now boast celiac disease centers.[68] Five national organizations disseminate information about the disease to patients, physicians, and the general public, seek increased funding for research, help celiacs manage their condition, and advocate on their behalf. Celiac support groups have proliferated throughout the country. And approximately two dozen drug treatments for celiac are in various stages of development. The growth of social media coincided with and undoubtedly contributed to the rise in celiac awareness. The Pew Research Center first began to track social media usage in 2005, two years after Fasano alerted the medical profession to the high prevalence of celiac in the United States. At that time 7 percent of American adults used social networking sites; ten years later, nearly two-thirds (65 percent) did.[69] People with celiac can learn about their disease from various social media sources, including message boards, the websites of advocacy organizations and celiac disease centers, and the various platforms of the many celiac influencers who offer advice while trying to shape purchasing decisions.

The following chapters demonstrate, however, that celiac has been slower to gain public and medical recognition than advocates originally anticipated. Because the level of knowledge among physicians remains low, many fail to diagnose the disease. Celiacs report that many friends, family members, and employers doubt the existence of the disorder and fail to understand the extreme measures sufferers must take to safeguard their health. Encountering derision and disbelief when they insist on rigorously following the gluten-free diet, some withdraw from all social activities.

2

Gluten-Free Food

Trivial Fad or Medical Necessity?

When I tell friends and colleagues that I am writing about celiac, many respond that this must be a good time to live with that disease. Walking down supermarket aisles, they see gluten-free food everywhere. But the popularity of the gluten-free diet has not been an unambiguous boon for the celiac community. Widespread publicity has helped to trivialize the diet as a fad and left all its adherents vulnerable to ridicule. Some gluten-free food items are now more appealing and available than ever before, but they remain expensive and unhealthy.

Although some food is naturally free of gluten (e.g., meat, potatoes, rice, vegetables, corn, and fruit), the term "gluten-free food" typically refers to processed items. Of course, most food is processed to at least some extent, if only to aid preservation. When people talk about processed food, they generally mean ultraprocessed foods (UPF), which contain numerous ingredients to make them more palatable (and often less nutritious). Nearly 60 percent of the calories Americans consume come in the form of UPF. Examples include hot dogs, boxed macaroni and cheese, frozen meals, and packaged baked goods.[1] The gluten-free market consists of many of the same products reformulated to eliminate wheat, barley, and rye. Peter H. R. Green, director of the Celiac Disease Center at Columbia University, notes that most of these gluten-free alternatives "are actually junk food. . . . Because what are the things that sell food? Salt, sugar, fat, and gluten. If the makers take one away, then they add more of another to keep it attractive to people."[2]

The Boom in Gluten-Free Food

Opening the doors to the Gluten Free Expo in Sandy, Utah, in November 2011, Debby Deaver anticipated attracting a small crowd. The weather was cold and rainy; Sandy was not well known; and most people associated gluten-free foods with the taste of cardboard. But four hundred people arrived in the first ten minutes, twelve hundred in the first hour, and six thousand by the end of the day. "They came from as far away as Arizona and Nebraska," wrote a *New York Times* reporter, "like pilgrims to a sort-of gluten free mecca."[3] The NPD group, a market-research company, found that one-third of Americans wanted to avoid or reduce gluten in their diet in 2013.[4] The following year NielsenIQ reported that 11 percent of households purchased gluten-free products, up 5 percent from 2010.[5] According to the *Wall Street Journal*, sales of items labeled gluten free more than doubled between 2010 and 2014.[6] Estimates of the size of the market vary widely, depending on the measure used. The research firm Mintel bases its estimate on all products labeled gluten free, including those that naturally are free of gluten. In 2013, it set the sales figure at $10.5 billion. By contrast, Euromonitor, which restricts its definition to products specifically reformulated to be gluten free, provided the much lower figure of $485.5 million. The two firms agreed, however, that the size of the market was increasing rapidly.[7]

As early as 2010, market researchers began to advise manufacturers that the gluten-free craze was on the verge of collapse. That year Suzy Badaracco, president of Culinary Tides, described the gluten-free market as "a house of cards just waiting to fall."[8] Four years later she stated, "Not only have we already hit the ceiling, the gluten-free bubble is already bursting and consumers are abandoning the diet." As a result, companies that had launched gluten-free products "are already recognizing that they might need an exit strategy."[9] In 2019, Gill Hyslop, editor of *BakeryandSnacks*, asked, "Is the gluten-free trend all just hype? Does gluten sensitivity really exist? Are more people being diagnosed with celiac disease? What will happen when the number of gluten-free consumers dwindle as they move on to the next big lifestyle?"[10] Despite such warnings, the gluten-free market has continued to flourish.[11]

The rise in the number of diagnoses of celiac disease can only partially explain this phenomenon. Celiac sufferers account for just 1 percent of the population, and many are unaware they are included in that group. People with nonceliac gluten sensitivity represent another 6–8 percent of the population. Thus, although 65 percent of the people who choose gluten-free food say they want to improve their health, most have neither condition.[12]

But Americans have long been preoccupied by the relationship between diet and health and became even more so after chronic disease began to replace acute illnesses as the major cause of death. As growing numbers of people began to realize that what they ate could affect their life expectancy, they started to search for healthier products. Moreover, dietary reformers increasingly embraced what American studies professor Warren Belasco called "Negative Nutrition." No longer encouraging Americans to eat more food, reformers began to point to different foods that should be eliminated or reduced.[13] The ingredients manufacturers added to improve the taste of processed food came under special attack. After five years of investigation, the US Senate Select Committee on Nutrition and Human Needs, led by Senator George McGovern, issued *Dietary Goals for the United States* in 1977. Introducing the report, McGovern stated, "Our diets have changed radically within the past fifty years, with great and often harmful effects on our health. . . . Too much fat, too much sugar, and salt, can be and are directly linked to heart disease, cancer, obesity, and stroke, among other killer diseases." Two years later the surgeon general's report *Healthy People* underlined that conclusion, calling on Americans to "emphasize the prevention of disease" by eating less fat, sugar, and salt.[14] The news about the evils of gluten thus reached a population already familiar with the notion that certain invisible ingredients could inflict serious damage.

The news also arrived at a time when neoliberalism was in the ascendance. In his 1981 inaugural address, President Ronald Reagan declared that "government is not the solution to our problems, government is the problem." That statement assumes that responsibility for health rests with individuals rather than the state. As Reagan's administration proceeded to dismantle various social programs, eating right and other lifestyle changes were accorded primacy while environmental and structural reforms increasingly lost support.[15]

Slightly more than a quarter (27 percent) of Americans say they avoid gluten to lose weight.[16] Because weight loss and health are so intimately connected in the popular mind, this may not represent an entirely different explanation. The US government certified that relationship in 2001 when it released *The Surgeon General's Call to Action to Prevent and Decrease Overweight and Obesity*, declaring that those conditions "have reached epidemic proportions in the United States." Although the nation had made "dramatic progress over the last few decades in achieving so many of our health goals," widespread overweight and obesity threatened to "wipe out the gains . . . in areas such as heart disease, diabetes, several forms of cancer, and other chronic health problems. Unfortunately, excessive weight for height is a risk factor for all of these conditions." The surgeon general added that weight loss was a "community responsibility" as well as a personal one. Children should have "safe, accessible" places to play; schools should require physical education and provide healthy food choices in their cafeterias; expectant mothers should be educated about the benefits of breastfeeding.[17]

Thinness also has a moral valence. "Despite ongoing debates about the probable causes and possible solutions of the epidemic," Charlotte Biltekoff writes, "the campaign against obesity consistently reinforced the social value of self-control. It insisted on an irrefutable equivalence between thinness and self-control that extended to an equivalence between thinness and fitness for citizenship."[18] Moreover, although large bodies were idealized in previous eras, slenderness now is widely considered essential to beauty. This is especially true for women, who are encouraged to aspire to a body size that is clinically underweight and unattainable for most. A survey of ten thousand women in the United States found that 85 percent wanted to be thinner.[19]

Popular ideas about fatness pervaded two books that helped to sound the alarm about gluten. In 2011, cardiologist William Davis published *Wheat Belly: Lose the Wheat, Lose the Weight, and Find Your Path Back to Health*, arguing that genetic modifications had made the wheat we consume far more dangerous than the product our ancestors ate. Modern wheat, he contended, contains numerous toxins, most notably gluten, which contributes to obesity. "As a cardiologist who saw and treated thousands of patients at risk for heart disease, diabetes, and the myriad destructive effects of obesity," he wrote, "I have personally observed protuberant, flop-over belt belly fat *vanish* when patients eliminated wheat from their diets. . . . Rapid and effortless weight loss is usually followed by health benefits that continue to amaze me even today after having witnessed this phenomenon thousands of times."[20] As this quotation indicates, Davis viewed overweight and obesity as unattractive as well as unhealthy. "Now put down that onion bagel," he instructed. "Your life, health, and appearance will never be the same."[21] Fat bodies disgusted him. Glancing at a photograph taken at the beach before he lost weight, he saw himself "fast asleep on the sand, my flabby abdomen splayed to either side, my second chin resting on my crossed flabby arms."[22] He recoiled from "people who waddle, limp, or ride scooters in XXL pants and dresses" and hoped to return his readers "to being slender, small-waisted . . . , not needing compressive clothing to conceal embarrassing body folds."[23] Like directors advertising weight-loss programs, Davis included before-and-after photographs of people who adhered to his regimen. Kathleen was "eighty pounds lighter after eighteen months grain-free." Niki "started at 224 pounds. Now, twelve months later," she weighed 178. And Keoni shed 60 pounds in fourteen months.[24]

Two years after *Wheat Belly* appeared, neurologist David Perlmutter followed with *Grain Brain: The Surprising Truth about Wheat, Carbs, and Sugar—Your Brain's Silent Killers*. "Gluten isn't just an issue for those with bona fide celiac disease," he asserted. "As many as 40 percent of us can't properly process gluten, and the remaining 60 percent could be in harm's way." Like Davis, he drew on his own experience, emphasized his surprise at his findings, and listed various conditions a gluten-free diet could alleviate: "Many of the individuals who reach out to me for guidance do so once they have 'tried everything' and have been to scores of other doctors in search of help." Regardless of which neurological disorder they present, one of his first actions is to "prescribe the total elimination of gluten from their diets." The results, he emphasized, "continue to amaze me." Autism, infertility, and schizophrenia were among the thirty-eight conditions he contended a gluten-free diet could prevent or alleviate.[25]

Self-control was an important theme in Perlmutter's book. His ideal audience consisted of people who acted with deliberation, and refused to yield to temptation. Now they must learn to "plan meals in advance," "prepare shopping lists," and "create a few 'non-negotiables.'" The last suggested that he assumed his readers had no overwhelming financial and time constraints: "If you have high hopes of getting to the farmers' market on Thursday afternoon in your neighborhood, then write that down in your calendar and make it a non-negotiable. If you dream of trying a new yoga studio that opened up in town, set aside a specific time and make it happen. Creating non-negotiable goals will help you dodge those excuses that surface when you get lazy or thwarted by other tasks. They are also excellent ways to fortify your weak spots. Be clear about your priorities." Perlmutter acknowledged that "a few indulgences" might be "inevitable" during holidays, but insisted that "as long as you get back on track once you catch yourself, you'll be fine. Just don't let a small slip derail you forever. To this end, remember to find consistency in your daily pattern."[26]

Scientists, food experts, and physicians quickly condemned both *Wheat Belly* and *Grain Brain*. Several critics noted that, contrary to Davis's contention, modern varieties of wheat do not contain more gluten than previous ones did.[27] Moreover, he based some of his conclusions on studies that no longer are considered credible.[28] An article in the *Ameri-*

can Journal of Cardiology argued that Perlmutter's "declaration that a single, simple 'cure' can successfully treat numerous diverse diseases and symptoms is reminiscent of the oratory of the 'snake oil' merchants of generations ago."[29] Most seriously, the argument of both authors that everyone can safely eat more high-cholesterol/fat products to replace grains flies in the face of scientific evidence. "There are certainly some people who are healthier with a higher-fat, lower-carbohydrate diet," commented Susan Roberts, director of the Energy Metabolism Laboratory at the Jean Mayer USDA Human Nutrition Research Center at Tufts, "but we have no evidence that this is more than a small percentage of the population."[30]

Although it was less often noted by critics, both books also made misleading comments about celiac disease. According to Davis, "The ways that celiac disease shows itself are . . . changing."[31] Both children and adults now have symptoms that differ from the ones celiac sufferers previously displayed. Davis acknowledges that "much of the changing face of celiac disease can certainly be attributed to earlier diagnosis aided by more reliable antibody blood tests." Once again, however, he finds the more probable cause in recent modifications of wheat. A more serious problem with his argument is that it ignores the fact that the celiac disease diagnosed today is a very different entity from the one earlier generations defined. Perlmutter exaggerates the prevalence of the disease. "Although many experts estimate that 1 in every 100 people worldwide has celiac disease," he wrote, "this is a conservative calculation; the number is probably closer to 1 in 30, since so many individuals remain undiagnosed." As already noted, however, the 1 percent figure includes undiagnosed patients as well as diagnosed ones. Perlmutter also asserted that "celiac disease is what happens when allergic reaction to gluten causes damage specifically to the small intestine."[32] Gastroenterologists define celiac as an autoimmune disease, not an allergy; thus gluten does not produce an "allergic reaction."

Despite those issues, the two books reached wide audiences, remaining on several bestseller lists for weeks. Like a long line of dietary reformers before them, Davis and Perlmutter promoted themselves shamelessly.³³ Although the gluten-free boom began before either book was published, both authors credited themselves with having launched it. The cover of the 2018 edition of *Grain Brain* boasted that the earlier edition "kick-started a revolution. Since then, it has been translated into thirty languages, and more than 1.5 million readers have been given the tools to make monumental improvements in their health." In his 2018 introduction, Perlmutter called his book "a global phenomenon," noting that he had given "countless" lectures around the world. "One of my most gratifying experiences occurred in 2017," he wrote, "when I shared my views on brain health at the World Bank, a presentation that was broadcasted on 150 sites around the planet."³⁴ Davis used equally hyperbolic language. The back cover of the second (2019) edition of *Wheat Belly* declared that the book had "introduced the world to the hidden dangers of modern wheat and gluten, revolutionizing the conversation around health and weight loss forever." His new foreword claimed that the previous edition had reached "millions of readers." Moreover, "Not eating this thing called wheat, celebrated by virtually all who offer dietary advice, is a revelation as big as recognizing that trafficking humans is a bad idea or that enslaving populations for cheap labor is not right."³⁵

People who read neither of those books could learn about the dangers of gluten in a host of other widely distributed publications and on health-related television shows. Recipes following Davis's and Perlmutter's suggestions appeared in both cookbooks and popular journals. The *New York Times* reported in 2011 that more than sixty gluten-free cookbooks had appeared in the previous year alone.³⁶ Celebrities added their endorsements. In 2010 singer Miley Cyrus declared that "everyone should try no gluten for a week! The change in your skin, physical and mental health is amazing! U won't go back!"³⁷ Others, including Jennifer Aniston, Kim Kardashian, Lady Gaga, and Victoria Beckham, claimed that a gluten-free diet was the key to both better health and weight loss.³⁸

Some evidence suggests that athletes were especially receptive to messages about gluten. An Australian study found that 41 percent of athletes adhered to some kind of gluten-free diet. Although the prevalence of gastrointestinal problems among members of this group is unusually high, the influence of the Serbian tennis player Novak Djokovic was also important.[39] In 2010 Djokovic underwent an extremely unusual and unscientific test for gluten sensitivity. A doctor asked him to hold out his right arm while placing his left hand on his stomach and then to stretch his right arm while holding a loaf of bread in his left hand. Because his arm was weaker the second time, the doctor convinced Djokovic that he had a gluten allergy. As he explained in his 2013 book, *Serve to Win*, his weight dropped but his strength increased when he restricted himself to a gluten-free diet.[40] (Djokovic is also an anti-vaxxer and was expelled from Australia for refusing to be vaccinated.)

The Costs of Publicity

The enormous publicity around gluten-free diet has not served celiacs well. The diet that is a medical necessity for them has been trivialized as a lifestyle choice. Even while some media outlets still were extolling the benefits of gluten-free diets, others began to label adherents as annoying, unmanly, overprivileged, or ridiculous. Cartoons in two widely circulated magazines had the same theme. The *New Yorker* cartoon featured two women eating together outside. One comments, "I've only been gluten free for a week but I'm already really annoying." Another *New Yorker* cartoon displayed three office workers holding out an empty plate to a fourth. One man explains, "We couldn't find a raw, vegan, gluten-free, sugar free, non-G.M.O. cake for your birthday, so we got you nothing."[41] *Elle* posted a cartoon on both Instagram and Facebook of a woman holding herself tightly while sitting in a large glass bowl. To her side are two women eating at a table, one of whom comments, "We get it, Amanda. You're gluten-free."[42] When Rachael Ray presented a "gluten-free" recipe in her magazine, she introduced it with a quotation linking gluten avoiders with other "picky eaters." (She also demonstrated her ignorance of gluten by including Corn Flakes in the recipe.)[43]

Newspapers published angry letters. "Why Do Your Kid's Allergies Mean My Kid Can't Have a Birthday?" was the headline of a 2014 article in the *HuffPost* Contributor platform. "I am rapidly reaching the end of my rope as I try to accommodate what feels like every child in the universe," the author wrote. "My children's school requires that we only provide store-bought treats because some children have allergies or dietary restrictions." She explained that she understood the problem with allergies because she herself was allergic to egg whites. "The difference is I don't demand egg-free items when I go to parties or to work events. I don't always get to eat what people are serving, but I certainly don't demand that my friend make a separate cake for me on her birthday." She concluded, "Let's stop the allergy insanity, and let the rest of them eat cake—the lovely, homemade, buttery, gluten-stuffed cake."[44] Three years later another woman complained to the *Washington Post* that restaurants that attempt to cater to everyone else's dietary restrictions curtail her own enjoyment. Sophie Egan was standing in the kitchen of Next Door, a casual chain restaurant in Stapleton, Colorado, when she realized that "food sensitivities are driving the culinary decision-making of entire operations: rather than jury-rigging dishes to respond to special needs, chefs have engineered many menus from the start to eschew everything from soy to gluten. And most customers don't have a clue." She had not minded when pizza places offered gluten-free crust to those who needed it or when a waiter asked if anyone had any food intolerances. But here was a restaurant that was "equally friendly to gluten-free, vegetarian, vegan, and various food-allergic customers as it is to everybody else." It suddenly dawned on her: "The afflictions of the minority are starting to determine the options for the majority."[45]

Despite the large number of athletes who proclaim themselves gluten free, people who choose that diet also are portrayed as unmanly. In NASCAR's 2015 Super Bowl ad, the actor Nick Offerman declared, "When our idea of danger is eating gluten, there's trouble afoot. Yes, we the people have gotten soft."[46] Four years later a *Barstool Sports* ad called those who avoid gluten "weak" and "pathetic."⁴⁷ A May 2013 episode of the Disney Channel show *Jessie* joked about a boy named Stuart who said he could not eat gluten. When another child threw a pancake at him, he screamed and wiped his face. A third boy said, "He makes me look macho."⁴⁸ As a presidential candidate in 2016, Senator Ted Cruz criticized President Barack Obama for "seven years of neglect" of the US military. Arguing that the country needed to "prioritize a strong, advanced, and robust military," he promised that it would not provide gluten-free meals.⁴⁹ Appearing on the NBC News morning show *Today*, Joy Behar said she would not be attracted by a date who asked whether a particular food contained gluten. Although the co-anchor, Hoda Kotb, repeatedly pointed out that some people eliminated gluten for medical reasons, Behar insisted that she liked a "guy" who "devoured" his meat and then asked if she was going to eat hers, not one who was so fussy about what he ate.⁵⁰

Others describe people who eliminate gluten as rich and white. In a discussion with other filmmakers about Black resistance and racial justice, Sabaah Folayan commented that her 2018 debut, *Whose Streets*, directed with Damon Davis, taught viewers about "direct action, militarization, the media, police violence, children's roles in the movement. But if you're going to wait until someone dies to learn about it and then as soon as things cool off it's back to Frappuccinos and gluten-free this, that, and a third, we're going to be here over and over and over again."⁵¹ In 2020, lawyer Jaaye Person-Lynn told a newscaster that African Americans in Los Angeles increasingly were protesting in the wealthy, white communities on the west side: "We're going to start hitting those farmers' markets, right where people are most comfortable. While they are buying their gluten-free bread and their organic tomatoes, they're going to have to feel it the same way we do."⁵² In a 2015 *Saturday Night Live* show, three African American men discuss the changes gentrification has wrought in their neighborhood. One chides another, "You're acting like someone put gluten in your muffin."⁵³ Jimmy Kimmel, the host of *Jimmy Kimmel Live*, asserted that most Los Angelenos try not to eat gluten because "someone in their yoga class told them not to." (When he sent an interviewer to ask four non–gluten eaters to define gluten and none could, the audience roared with laughter.)[54] There is some truth to these characterizations. As we have seen, white, middle- and upper-class people are especially likely to receive celiac diagnoses. They also are more likely than others to buy gluten-free food, at least in part because it is more expensive than the alternative and more frequently available in their neighborhoods. A 2019 study of people who searched for the gluten-free diet on Google were disproportionately non-Hispanic whites with high incomes.[55]

We also can understand other reasons why the gluten-free diet provokes derision and exasperation. As already noted, food fads, often backed by scientific pronouncements, periodically have swept the country since the 1890s.[56] Derogatory comments about gluten-free-diet followers occasionally allude to that history. After learning that a longtime friend suddenly had decided to renounce gluten, David Klimas, a real estate sales manager, remarked, "I don't get it. How can you all of a sudden be gluten-free? He's 45. We've been friends for 19 years. Sometimes, I think it's just for him to be cool in front of the waiters." Klimas added, "In the '50s, everyone had ulcers. Then, it was back problems. Now, it's gluten."[57] Journalist Jeffrey Kluger predicted that "eventually, the gluten-free cookbooks will wind up in the same river of pop detritus as the no-carb wines and the fat-free cookies and the crock pots and fondue sets and woks everyone in America seemed to buy at once in 1988 and stopped using sometime around 1989."[58]

The casualness with which some people without medical diagnoses treat the gluten-free diet contributes to the notion that it is a trivial fad. Jessie Dankos, a twenty-four-year-old grant-management consultant in Virginia, complained about her roommate, who wanted sympathy for refusing to indulge in baked goods when dining out but then occasionally ate a slice of pizza at home.[59] In that context, celiac sufferers who insist that even the smallest bread crumb can inflict harm begin to seem excessively preoccupied with their health.

Restaurants are one place where frivolous requests can have serious repercussions. "After witnessing enough diners who make a big fuss about how their bodies can't tolerate gluten and then proceed to order a beer or dig into their dates' brownie dessert," Neil Swidey writes, "fatigued chefs and managers are beginning to adopt a less accommodating approach."[60] In an extreme but widely publicized example, a former banquet chef at the Tavern on the Green in Central Park posted this on his Facebook page:

> Gluten free is bullshit!! Flour and Bread have been a staple of life for thousands, THOUSANDS of years. People who claim to be gluten intolerant don't realize that its [sic] all in there [sic] disturbed little heads. People ask me for gluten free pasta in my restaurants all the time, I tell em sure. Then I serve em our pasta. Which I make from scratch with high gluten flour. And you know what? Nothing, NOTHING! Ever happens! People leave talking about how good they feel gluten free and guess what. They just had a full dose! Idiots![61]

What he failed to understand, of course, was that guests with celiac disease would not have an immediate response; symptoms of having been "glutened" typically would occur hours after they left the restaurant.

The large number of diners who claim allergies exacerbates the situation. Swidey asked numerous chefs what proportion of their tables include at last one person demanding the elimination of certain ingredients on a typical night. The estimates ranged from 10 to 60 percent. When the requests reach a kitchen "crammed with cooks and dishwashers," Swidey continues, the action stops while the cooks "consult a printed breakdown of ingredients in each dish. They either grab new cutting boards, knives, tongs or put theirs through the sanitizing dishwasher. And when the plate is done, they use disposable wipes to hold it by the edge."[62] As we will see, celiac sufferers complain that only a tiny fraction of restaurants take such precautions and eating out remains exceedingly dangerous in most places. Nevertheless, Swidey's account highlights the consequences of large numbers of people without medical conditions insisting on special accommodations. When a restaurant that prided itself on its gluten-free offerings gave a woman gluten-containing bread by mistake, she complained on the celiac.com forum, "so frustrated that the restaurant obviously decided I was gluten-free to be trendy and didn't really have a health issue" (June 23, 2015).

The celiac community has responded to the trivialization of the gluten-free diet by pointing out that it is no joke to them. After the late-night talk show host Jimmy Fallon elicited cheers and laughter by calling the gluten-free cookbook his guest had written "garbage" and then smashing a pie on the author's face, Priyanka Chugh, a gastroenterologist and celiac blogger, posted an open letter that read in part, "Mr. Fallon, you make light of the fact that eating gluten can make us ill. There's a term for that. It's called ableism, and according to Merriam-Webster, it's defined as 'discrimination or prejudice against individuals with disabilities.' When you take your place of privilege, as someone able-bodied, and use it to make jokes against those of us who are differently-abled, you are, in fact, participating in a form of social prejudice. When I put it in those terms, it really stops being funny, doesn't it."[63] Explaining why she started a Change.org petition demanding that Disney remove the offensive episode of *Jessie* from the air, a mother wrote,

> For my kids, this is real. They have had friends make fun of their food, been disinvited to parties because of their diet. They have been made to sit alone, have had waitstaff roll their eyes and snidely comment about their requests to make their food safe for them to eat. They have watched others, sometimes strangers and sometimes not, act as if their requests are somehow just a trend, just a request of an overanxious parent or a spoiled or coddled child. . . . Yet Disney gave children permission, and an example, to further isolate my children and others like them because of their medical conditions. Their characters made it okay to characterize a real illness as an annoyance that is justification for the "cool kids"

to make fun of the "others." This isn't acceptable for anyone. It is the definition of bullying.[64]

After the woman sent her petition, Disney pulled the episode.[65]

A few other protests also have achieved at least partial success. In response to a petition with fifteen thousand signatures protesting the NASCAR ad, NBC Sports eliminated Offerman's sentence from the spot that ran during the Super Bowl (though not from online versions).[66] Although the *Today Show* failed to apologize for the insults to gluten-free dieters on Hoda Kotb's program, it did post several angry responses from viewers on its Facebook page.[67] Gluten Dude provided an update of *Elle*'s gluten-free cartoon: "So after 9 hours of getting SLAMMED by the celiac community (take a bow folks), *Elle* has completely removed the post from both their Instagram and Facebook accounts. . . . Seen by millions and yet no acknowledgement. No apology. Such turds. Like it never existed. At least it's gone."[68]

Costs and Benefits

Examining Americans' relationship to food can help us understand both the advantages and disadvantages of the explosion of the market in processed gluten-free foods for celiacs. Various studies find that the factors Americans consider when making choices about purchasing food include health, price, taste, and convenience (though not necessarily in that order).[69]

Health

Despite the widespread assumption that gluten-free food promotes physical and mental well-being, most items are less healthy than traditional ones. They have lower levels of fiber, some micronutrients, and protein, and higher levels of fat, salt, and sugar. Various producers have experimented with enhancing the nutritional value of gluten-free food, but studies find that celiacs have nutritional deficiencies not only at the time of diagnosis but also while on the gluten-free diet. Although celebrities boast of the pounds they shed after avoiding gluten, many gluten-free products have higher caloric content than their wheat-based counterparts and thus lead to weight gain.[70] Studies finding high levels of arsenic in rice have raised additional concerns.[71]

As a result, many doctors caution people unaffected by either celiac or nonceliac gluten sensitivity not to restrict themselves to gluten-free food. Alessio Fasano, the physician who did more than anyone else to spread awareness of celiac disease and the consequent need for a gluten-free diet, remarked in 2015, "We did such a good job that the monster went all out of control."[72] The Canadian Celiac Association, the American Heart Association, the Obesity Society, and the American College of Cardiology have all refused to endorse gluten-free diets for anyone without celiac disease or gluten intolerance.[73]

Convenience

Most Americans look for ways to reduce the time and effort required to put food on the table.[74] The greater availability of gluten-free food items has made shopping for them easier. In 2014, CBS reported, "When Alice Bast was diagnosed with celiac disease in 1994, she had to scour local health-food stores and send away to Canada for the gluten-free food her condition necessitated." Two decades later celiacs could find "gluten-free choices much closer to home—in the way of takeout from the Chinese restaurant down the street, options at the local supermarket, and on the shelves of a nearby CVS."[75]

But scrutinizing food labels takes time many people cannot afford.[76] "Having celiac disease can feel like a full-time job all by itself," wrote actress Jennifer Esposito. "Take going to the market. It's not happening in less than an hour because you have to read every label and look at every single thing you put in your cart, especially when you're new at it." With full-time television work in addition to searching for something to eat, Esposito felt "truly overwhelmed."[77] Celiacs who are unsure about the safety of a particular product are advised to phone manufacturers, a practice one celiac.com forum participant described as "very frustrating and time consuming" (April 15, 2010). Moreover, as we will see, a significant fraction of celiacs live in food deserts. Without access to supermarkets, they rely on convenience stores and fast-food restaurants that offer little, if any, gluten-free food.

Flavor

In 2011, a *New York Times* article asserted, "A few years ago, tough and tasteless baked goods were just one of the unpleasant things you had to put up with if you had a gluten sensitivity."[78] Moreover, the products spoiled easily and were either too moist or too dry. Companies experimented with various ingredients to overcome these problems. For many, it was a matter of trial and error. Dean Creighton, a General Mills food scientist for more than two decades, "tinkered with cereal recipes" to reformulate Chex. Jodi Benson, another GM employee, noted that it was even more difficult to produce gluten-free baked goods. The early cake recipes fell flat. "Think of a yellow cake in a brownie height," Benson said. The team made a thousand batches before concluding that the new product was acceptable.[79] Despite similar efforts by other manufacturers, most people continue to find gluten-free items less appealing than other food.[80]

Cost

Columbia University researchers found that between 2006 and 2016, the cost of gluten-free products compared to their wheat-based counterparts declined from 240 percent to 183, still a significant burden to anyone on a tight budget.[81] We will see that several celiac.com participants complained that the expense of gluten-free food was prohibitive for them.

Cooking as an Alternative

Given the many disadvantages of processed gluten-free food (especially with regard to cost and health), we may wonder why more celiacs do not prepare their meals from basic ingredients that are naturally free of gluten. Doctors and nutritionists advise newly diagnosed people to avoid all processed food while they are trying to heal and consume them sparingly, if at all, thereafter. The proliferation of cookbooks enables them to do so. In January 2023 Amazon has 949 entries for "celiac disease cookbooks" and more than 1,000 entries for "gluten free cookbooks best sellers 2022." Beginners as well as experienced cooks can learn how to prepare gluten-free meals in a hurry or for special occasions. They can become bakers, producing gluten-free alternatives to almost all the store-brought goods they no longer can eat. They can use slow cookers or instant pots, feed both children and adults, and learn how to serve those who are not only gluten free but also diabetic, lactose intolerant, or vegan.

But most people want food that is familiar.[82] The first thing many celiacs do after receiving a diagnosis is try to replace familiar foods that suddenly are forbidden. "Everybody (including myself) is told to eat plain whole foods at first," one woman wrote to the celiac.com forum, "and everybody (including myself) goes right out and buys gluten-free substitutes right away any way. I think it's because we feel so deprived at first and want our daily bread" (November 5, 2015). The addictive quality of most processed food compounds the sense of deprivation. "Most of us can't simply stop eating processed foods," Michael Moss writes, explaining that our taste buds have been "jacked up" to desire the high levels of salt, sugar, and fat the products contain.[83]

Moreover, massive marketing campaigns overwhelm whatever dietary advice celiacs receive from medical professionals. A 2022 report issued by the World Health Organization contained few surprises when it concluded that food marketing in general "has been shown to impact strongly on food preferences and consumption patterns." Because celiac disease is often diagnosed in childhood, findings about the harmful effects of ads targeting children are especially significant. The report continued, "Children in particular have been identified as being particularly susceptible to the messages used in marketing communications and it is now widely acknowledged that exposure to food marketing is a risk factor for the development of childhood obesity."[84]

Noting that 30 percent of Americans said that they try to reduce the amount of gluten they eat, Harry Balzer, vice president of the NPD Group, remarked in 2014, "If you find 30 percent of the public doing anything, you'll find a lot of marketers right there, too."[85] Subsequent chapters demonstrate that gluten-free food marketing directed to celiacs takes various forms. The major celiac advocacy organizations solicit sponsorships from food companies and promote their products. Celiac influencers on social media earn money by reviewing different brands and writing recipes that incorporate them. At the many gluten-free-food expositions held throughout the country, manufacturers have booths where they sell their products and give away free samples.

Finally, exhortations to cook at home oppose long-term trends. The amount of time Americans spend in the kitchen each day dropped from three hours in the 1920s to two in the late 1960s. By the 1990s, the time had fallen to one hour and by 2013 to half of that.[86] In 2019, Americans spent more than half (54 percent) of their food budget on items prepared away from home.[87] Laura Shapiro argues that some of the decline in domestic cooking resulted from food-industry pressure. Having invented various kinds of processed food to feed the troops in World War II, the industry launched a massive campaign to convince women that cooking was a chore they should be happy to relinquish. "Magazines, newspapers, and radio announcers," Shapiro writes, "explained over and over to housewives that a welcome new era of effortless food preparation was at hand. 'You don't cook it,' promised an ad for Sunkist lemons, brandishing a recipe for making lemon pie in an ice cube tray. 'Just mix and beat as directed, place in the refrigerator—*and that's all.*'"[88] Just as the food industry today tries to persuade people with celiac to rely on processed food products, so it previously sought to convince women that they hated to cook and that packaged, frozen, and canned items were superior to their own concoctions.

More recently, the decline in the amount of time spent in the kitchen coincided with an increase in working hours. In her 1992 book, *The Overworked American*, economist Juliet B. Schor estimated that the average American put in 163 more hours a year than she or he had in 1973.[89] Today, Americans work 14 percent more hours per year than Europeans, at least in part because the United States lags far behind in providing basic job protections.[90] People who cannot afford gluten-free food are thus least likely to be able to cook for themselves and their families.

Even before Schor's book appeared, sociologists began to report that unpaid domestic work meant especially long hours for women. Although housework is now distributed more equitably between the genders, the burden continues to fall more heavily on women.[91] Any increase in the time spent on cooking adds to that burden.

"We can make delicious and nutritious food at home," Georgianne wrote on the celiac.com forum, "but we need to learn how to cook and how to take gluten-free safety measures, and let's face it, if you have two jobs and kids, you can't cook everything you eat no matter how resourceful you are" (July 22, 2005). Other forum participants cited competing obligations to explain why they did not prepare more of their own food. "With 2 really small kids (2 yrs and 9 months)," Ruby was "having a hard time making time to cook every meal" (November 5, 2016). Steven wrote, "Seems many gluten-free people have to go right back to basics and cook everything from scratch. That's a problem for me as I'm utterly hopeless on that front and time doesn't permit waiting hours just to prepare one meal. Seems nigh-on impossible to do day-in, day out" (June 15, 2016). Anne, a college student, had a job in addition to her school work, "so I don't have a whole lot of time to spend cooking" (March 26, 2018). One of the few writers who prepared most of her meals herself, Jessica had little time left for other activities. "I really do enjoy cooking," she wrote.

However, I find myself feeling like I live in my kitchen. I really love gardening and haven't had time to do that anymore along with a bunch of other things. . . . I used to be one of those people who would throw a last minute meal together or stop by and pick up Chinese or go to the salad bar or meet friends for dinner. Now, I don't do any of those things anymore. I am not necessarily complaining, it just seems that this is all so time consuming and unfortunate that I have had to give up things due to the time I spend cooking. (June 15, 2011)

Conclusion

Although the phenomenal growth of the gluten-free food market has enormous implications for people with celiac, it did not stem from a recognition of their needs and does not always benefit them. Because most processed gluten-free products contain even more fat, salt, and sugar than their wheat-based counterparts and have less nutritional value, the items are especially inappropriate for people who have difficulty absorbing nutrients and must exercise special care about their health. Most products are prohibitively expensive for those on low incomes. We will see that symptoms force many celiacs out of the labor force, further limiting their ability to purchase costly food. As the gluten-free diet has become less newsworthy, followers are less likely to encounter mockery and irritation. Nevertheless, celiacs continue to complain about the difficulty of explaining why they must take such extreme care to adhere to a diet that other people treat far more casually.

3

Is It Really Gluten Free?

Clarifying the Claims

Although reports of the unhealthiness of processed foods encourage some celiacs to avoid them entirely, it is almost impossible for most people to do so. As a result, celiacs must rely on front-of-packaging labeling (FOPL) to learn whether packaged food products contain unacceptable amounts of gluten. But FOPL has long been mired in controversy. "The history of nutritional labels in modern times is a game of cat and mouse between researchers, regulatory agencies, and food manufacturers," wrote the MIT Center for Civic Media. "The general pattern of the 20th century appears to have consisted of food companies free to sell most anything until a major outcry, poisoning, or exposé leads to new regulation."[1] The food industry has waged a long battle against regulations to clarify the meaning of "gluten free" on product labels; in response, celiac advocates have fought to increase transparency in food marketing.

Food Allergen Labeling and Consumer Protection Act

When the Nutrition Labeling and Education Act, the first major food-label law, was passed in 1990, neither allergies nor celiac disease had begun to receive attention from health professionals. Awareness of allergies came first.[2] (Unlike celiac disease, food allergies cause immediate adverse reactions; the most serious, anaphylactic shock, can be fatal. The eight major allergens are milk, egg, fish, shellfish, nuts, wheat, and soybeans.)

Long after Clemens von Pirquet, an Austrian pediatrician, coined the term "allergy" in 1906, doctors knew little about the phenomenon. Conflicts between physicians who diagnosed and treated allergic patients and allergists in academic and laboratory settings contributed to the marginalization of the field. Reports of a growing number of fatalities from anaphylactic shock, however, served to galvanize parents into action.[3] The *New York Times* reported one tragedy in 1986. Kate Brodsky was an eighteen-year-old Brown University student when she died after eating a few spoonfuls of chili thickened with peanut butter in a restaurant. "She had known she was allergic to nuts since she was 2 or 3," her mother commented. "She couldn't stand the smell of peanuts and she consciously avoided any food that had nuts in it. Who would expect peanut butter in chili?" The article continued, "Doctors know surprisingly little about food allergies. They do not know, for example, how best to test for food allergies, how to treat them or why some people are allergic to foods and others are not. They can say for certain, however, that severe allergic reactions, like the one Miss Brodsky suffered, are rare."[4]

Although anaphylactic incidents are extremely uncommon, they enabled parents to publicize the dangers all food allergies posed. In 1991, Anne Muñoz-Furlong, whose daughter had been diagnosed with allergies to milk and eggs as a young child, organized the Food Allergy Network (later the Food Allergy and Anaphylaxis Network [FAAN]) to increase public awareness of food allergies.[5] A prolific writer, Muñoz-Furlong placed articles in popular publications and soon received supportive letters from other parents. In a newsletter, *Food Allergy News*, and on the Internet, she offered both scientific information and practical advice about living with food allergies. In addition, her group produced booklets for parents, teachers, and children with such titles as "Off to School with Food Allergies," "Understanding Food Labels," and the "Nutritional Guide to Food Allergies." Children with allergies were offered laminated cards with instructions about reading food labels. A program called "Be a Pal" sought to educate other children about the dangers their allergic classmates faced.[6] Gradually schools, day care centers, and summer camps began to take precautions.[7] "While it is unclear whether the number of people with allergies is on the rise," the *New York Times* wrote in 1998," awareness of their needs certainly is."[8]

As news about the severity and prevalence of food allergies spread, activists increasingly focused on FOPL inadequacies. Studies identified several problems. Although the food industry was required to list all ingredients by their "common or usual" names, some companies employed such terms as "albumin," "lecithin," "livetin," "lysozyme," "emulsifier," "globulin," "ovalbumin," and "vitellin" for egg and such words as "caramel color," "casein," "caseinate," "high protein flavor," "albumin," "solids," and "whey" for milk. A 2002 study found that half of all parents with children with peanut allergies could not identify peanuts on labels.[9] In addition, labels were often incomplete. A 2000 survey of the members of FAAN reported that 98 percent indicated that food labels did not include enough information to enable them to make safe decisions. "Our members are some of the best educated, highly motivated people in the food allergy community and this country," commented Muñoz-Furlong. "If they are struggling with these labels, I can only imagine what the general public is going through."[10] A study sponsored by the Food and Drug Administration (FDA) and reported in the *New York Times* in 2001 found that 25 percent of manufacturers in Minnesota and Wisconsin produced items containing such allergens as peanuts but did not list them on package labels.[11] Advocates also noted that such words as "natural flavors," "artificial flavors," and "spices" commonly concealed allergens. The advisory warnings (such as "may contain X allergen" or "processed on shared equipment"), which manufacturers placed on labels to protect themselves from liability, were useless to consumers. And labels failed to indicate when items that were free of allergens became contaminated by them during the production process.[12]

In 2000, Representative Nita M. Lowey, a New York Democrat, introduced the Food Allergen Labeling and Consumer Protection Act (FALCPA), addressing some, but not all, of those issues. Soon afterwards, Senator Edward M. Kennedy introduced similar legislation in the Senate. Lowey later said that her motivation came from her many constituents who "had food allergies and had a hard time avoiding foods that could cause reactions because of unclear or inexact labeling."[13]

Opposition arose quickly from the food industry. Attempting to stave off legislative mandates, the industry issued voluntary guidelines in 2001. "Allergens are a major food industry priority," declared Alison Kretser, director of scientific and nutrition policy at the Grocery Manufacturers of America, one of the trade groups responsible for drafting the guidelines. She emphasized that they went "beyond federal regulations to meet the needs of allergic consumers."[14] The FDA praised the guidelines as "a significant step forward" and a "major health benefit to the food-allergy consumer." Muñoz-Furlong commended them for making "life safer for individuals with food allergies and their families."[15]

But compliance was inconsistent, and trade associations had no enforcement mechanism.[16] As the *New York Times* reported, "Kraft tells shoppers that whey comes from milk in Chips Ahoy cookies but makes no mention of that on boxes of Stove Top stuffing. Pillsbury's Moist Supreme Cake mix warns that the ingredients may accidently contain traces of egg but does not note that the 'whey proteins' it deliberately adds are from milk."[17] Lowey remarked, "It's just not enough to completely and accurately label some of the food some of the time. Too many bad food labels are still slipping through the cracks."[18] In a similar vein, a representative of the Center for Science in the Public Interest stated in a public meeting that "the time has long passed for all this total voluntary flexible action on the part of industry."[19]

Although groups for people with food allergies took the lead in campaigning for FALCPA, celiac advocates slowly became involved. As already noted, celiac still was considered a rare disease when Lowey and Kennedy first introduced the legislation. Medical professionals began to acknowledge the importance of the disorder only after 2003, when Alessio Fasano, an Italian gastroenterologist and medical director of the Center for Celiac Research at the University of Maryland, published a paper in the *Archives of Internal Medicine* demonstrating that celiac was far more common than previously assumed. That year Fasano founded the American Celiac Task Force (later the American Celiac Disease Alliance). The members included other researchers, leaders of advocacy organizations, and a few representatives of manufacturers of gluten-free food.[20] Interviewed in 2005, the cochair, Andrea Levario, commented that although the group had no money, it became an important "voice" in the campaign.[21]

Lowey made it clear that, despite the bill's title, her intent was to protect individuals with celiac disease as well as those with food allergies. After a mother and son testified before a congressional committee about the needs of people with celiac, Lowey explained that she had drafted her bill to help them.[22] Urging her colleagues to pass the bill a few months later, she again stated, "Navigating insufficient labels is much more than an irritation for the millions with food allergies. It is a matter of life and death. Unfortunately, the situation is the same for those with Celiac Disease, a lifelong digestive disorder that damages the small intestine and interferes with absorption of nutrients from food."[23] By that date, however, her bill no longer required manufacturers to disclose the presence of gluten on labels. Addressing the Senate in May 2002, Kennedy, chair of the Health, Education, Labor, and Pension Committee, commented that the law "will require that food ingredient statements on food packages identify in common language when an ingredient, including flavoring, coloring, or other additive, is itself, or is derived from, one of the eight main food allergens, or from grains containing gluten."[24] (Although wheat was one of the eight major allergens and therefore would be covered in the law, Kennedy indicated that the law also should include requirements for rye and barley.) But that September he worked out a compromise with the Republican members of his committee who supported the contention of the food industry that gluten was not an allergen. According to the report of the Food and Drug Administration on September 27, 2002, Kennedy's committee "passed without objection a watered down version of a bill that would require food processors to label the eight most common types of food allergens in plain English. The substitute version, unlike the underlying bill, would . . . not require the declaration of gluten."[25] That version became the basis for the law that finally was passed in 2004 and went into effect in 2006.

Andrea Levario later noted that she had welcomed the law because "eighty percent of the problem [for people with celiac disease] is in wheat or a wheat derivative."[26] Others, however, were less pleased. Laura E. Derr, a lawyer, explained that the labeling of wheat under the law "in fact, may have the perverse effect of harming those who must avoid gluten. A gluten-free product always is wheat-free, but the reverse is not true. Children or caregivers of children with celiac disease may assume incorrectly that a wheat-free product is gluten-free if they are not familiar with or do not remember the various terms for gluten-containing ingredients . . . besides wheat."[27]

Unsurprisingly, celiacs, too, expressed disappointment. "The labels will note the presence of wheat, and that is extremely helpful," one commented. "Yet without including the term gluten, the legislation falls short of allowing me to feel totally empowered. I will still have to call manufacturers to ensure that the products I buy do not contain any gluten."[28] The labeling also confused participants on the celiac.com forum. Carole recently had received a diagnosis. "I have begun to notice that several items say wheat free and make no mention of gluten," she wrote. "However, through some investigating on a Newman's Cookie box, I noticed that it said 'Wheat Free, not gluten free.' Is this the universal answer? Is it safe to assume that complex foods (those with more than 2 ingredients) should say 'gluten free' if they are? Help!" (May 14, 2008). The label on a product Maureen bought did indicate it was gluten free, but in much smaller letters than the ones declaring it wheat free. She had been delighted to find cookies that looked like Oreos in the supermarket aisle where she often found gluten-free food: "Yummmmmm! In big letters it said 'Wheat Free/Dairy Free.' Great, says I. Bought them. Took them home. Ate three. Sigh. So of course when I went back to read the label—after realizing that my reaction couldn't have been from the roast chicken—I saw the words, in little print, 'this is *not* a gluten-free food'" (July 13, 2010).

The act had other limitations as well. Most seriously, because it applied only to packaged foods, it did not cover medications and restaurants. As we will see in chapter 7, eating out has remained a major source of inadvertent gluten ingestion. The act also failed to directly address the issue of foods that were originally free of allergens but became contaminated during production. And it provided no guidance about the use of allergen warnings (such as "may have been processed in equipment shared with wheat").[29] Studies report that those warnings do not undermine gluten-free claims.[30] Nevertheless, the celiac.com forum indicates that celiacs remain concerned. One participant wrote, "At the store recently I found a bag of chips that had the 'certified gluten free' stamp on the front. I didn't even look at the back of the bag because of that stamp. A few days later I go to open the bag of chips and notice on the back that there's a disclaimer about the chips being produced in a facility that processes wheat. WHAT? Is this a thing? I'm new to being celiac but I thought that the certified stamp meant I could 100% trust the product. Just wondering if this kind of perplexing labeling is normal and is the food OK to eat?" (March 17, 2016). Lorna had a similar experience and was equally irate: "I just bought a big old box of trail mix packages from Sam's Club (first time shopping in there with the kids since diagnosis). It had GLUTEN FREE written all over the box, and it's all over each individual package, but when I got home and looked closer at the box it says manufactured on shared equipment with wheat!!! How can they have the GLUTEN FREE labeling all over it when it's been on shared equipment?" (April 13, 2017).

Developing Standards

FALCPA did not ignore the issue of gluten entirely. The Secretary of Health and Human Services was directed to propose a rule to define the term "gluten free" within two years and to issue a final rule within four. The Food and Drug Administration (FDA), the agency responsible for establishing the standard, met neither deadline.

Although celiac advocates came late to the campaign for passage of FALCPA, they participated actively in efforts to define "gluten free" from the beginning. "The celiac community is very tight," Fasano later commented, "and they followed this process every step of the way over the course of 10 years of meetings and public forums. The community always showed up big time to give their opinion."[31] In response to an FDA announcement of a public meeting in 2005 to discuss various approaches to setting a standard, the agency received more than twenty-four hundred comments, "the vast majority," according to the *Federal Register*, from people with celiac disease, their caregivers, and celiac advocacy organizations. "Many consumers stated that a 'gluten-free' labeling claim makes it easier to shop for groceries, saving the consumers both time and the frustration experienced when reading often lengthy and complicated ingredients lists that the consumers do not understand."[32]

In 2007, the FDA finally proposed that products could be labeled gluten free if ingredients containing gluten (wheat, barley, and rye) represented no more than twenty ppm (parts per million). The proposed rule did not please everyone. The Celiac Sprue Association (later Beyond Celiac), a consumer advocacy group, had argued that products labeled gluten free should contain no gluten because sensitive patients could not tolerate even the smallest amount. "We need to find testing that is meaningful, verifiable and consistent no matter what the product is and something that is durable during the entire manufacturing process," stated Mary Schluckebier, executive director of the association. She added, "I haven't seen any proposals [by the FDA] on good ways to absolutely ensure there is no cross contamination."[33] The International Wheat Gluten Association wanted a threshold of two hundred ppm.[34] Sukh Bassi, vice president for research and development of MGP Ingredients, a member of that association, argued that any gluten-free message was wrong. "It just scares people, makes them think gluten is a bad thing," he said.[35] But twenty ppm was the lowest level at which gluten could be detected; Canada and the European Union already had established that threshold, and most US food experts agreed it was appropriate.[36] The FDA asked for comments and launched a safety assessment.

And then nothing happened. While the gluten-free market exploded, the FDA failed to act. Consumers affected by celiac had no way of knowing whether the products they bought contained any gluten and, if so, how much. In February 2011 Max wrote on the celiac.com forum, "Just curious what others do when they've checked a manufacturer's list, found a 'gluten free' product, gone to purchase it only to find it has wheat in several identifiable components. Obviously, eating it is out of the question" (February 6, 2011). Thomas wrote the following month,

> I really, really find myself getting more and more frustrated by the term "gluten free," I think because it feels like such a deceptive term, honestly. Most of the doctors I talk to think it means zero gluten. Most of the people who are not celiacs I talk to think it means zero gluten. About a quarter of the company representatives I talk to about their gluten free products think it means zero gluten. And many of us start out thinking it means zero gluten, too. We start our diet, we look at our foods, and we always ask, "Is this gluten free?" If it has no gluten, then it must be safe, right? If this is 100% gluten free, then it's fine for us to eat. And that's so not true. . . .
>
> We have no law that is in effect in the USA, so all companies who use the term "gluten free" for their products are on the honor system. . . . It just feels like this label, while trying to help us, has caused potential issues as well. . . . How many of us *absolutely trusted* that gluten free label until the first time we got sick on an ostensibly gluten free product? It just feels like this label, while trying to help us, has also caused potential issues as well. (March 27, 2011)

By that spring, celiac advocates, too, had begun to express growing frustration. Levario noted that thousands of people affected by the disease had sent letters to the FDA demanding action but received no reply.[37] Alessio Fasano wrote, "The FDA has spent years calling upon experts to have open-forum debates, town hall meetings, we've been having reiteration and reiteration. They've been reiterating and listening to Grandma, Grandpa, people on the street corners. . . . I really don't understand why it's lingering up in the air when it really should be a no-brainer."[38] Other activists used a case decided in April to illustrate the dangers celiac sufferers continued to face. Paul Seelig was found guilty and sentenced to eleven years in prison for buying regular bread, repackaging it as gluten free, and then selling it through his North Carolina company, Great Specialty Products. Dozens of people became sick. "We thought it was fantastic because it tasted like regular bread," said Rebecca Fernandez, the mother of a two-year-old son with celiac. A bloody rash covered his body and he had diarrhea for weeks. "I called the police," she commented. "They said it wasn't really their thing." She then called the FDA's Charlotte office but received no reply. Finally, she contacted the North Carolina Department of Agriculture, which regulates bread in the state and conducted an investigation.[39] Zach Becker had recommended the company on his gluten-free Raleigh blog before he developed a blistering, bleeding rash from the bread. Appearing before the judge, he said that the lack of an FDA standard for gluten free "has left the gluten-free community vulnerable to fraudulent companies like Great Specialty Products."[40]

On May 4, a group of activists organized a Gluten-Free Food Labeling Summit in Washington, DC, to press the FDA to move forward. Attendees included legislators, researchers, gluten-free advocates, and representatives of food corporations. The conference opened with the display of a thirteen-foot gluten-free cake brought to Capitol Hill. "Doesn't it seem strange that Congress would have issued a mandate and years go by and it hasn't been done?" asked Jules Shepard, an organizer and gluten-free cookbook author. "It seems like the FDA is breaking the law, and it's time to do something about it."[41] Michael R. Taylor, FDA deputy commissioner for foods, assured the group that "we really understand that there's a big population out there and this is really a serious problem for them, and labeling can help and we want to do our part."[42]

A lawyer whose career illustrates the revolving door between government and industry, Taylor is a controversial figure. After receiving his

JD degree in 1976, he was a staff attorney for the FDA. Between 1981 and 1991, he worked at the large and prestigious law firm King and Spalding, representing the Monsanto Company, a major producer of chemical, agricultural, and biochemical products. He returned to the FDA in 1991 as deputy commissioner for policy; one of his major responsibilities was implementing the Nutrition Labeling and Education Act of 1990. Four years later Taylor received an appointment as administrator of the Food Safety and Inspection Service of the US Department of Agriculture. He rejoined King and Spalding in 1996, became vice president for public policy at Monsanto in 1998, and moved to the nonprofit think tank Resources for the Future in 2000. Obama appointed Taylor the senior advisor to the FDA in 2009. The following year he became the first person to hold the position of deputy commissioner for foods.[43]

Taylor's government career received mixed reports from consumers and advocates. Marion Nestle wrote that in his position as head of the Food Safety and Inspection Service in 1994, he "became the *hero* of food-safety activists for his courageous development of the agency's groundbreaking policies for controlling dangerous microbial contaminants in meat and industry." Three years earlier, however, he had played a role in issuing the FDA's "decidedly industry-friendly policy on food biotechnology" and in approving "the use of Monsanto's genetically engineered growth hormone in dairy cows."[44] Nestle's study ends before Taylor's appointment to the FDA in 2009, which ignited a storm of protests. One advocate wrote on his blog, "The person who may be responsible for more food-related illness and death than anyone in history has just been made the US food safety czar. This is no joke." A petition signed by tens of thousands of people soon after it was launched referred to Taylor as an example of a "fox watching the hen house."[45]

On July 21, 2011, two Democratic senators, Ron Wyden of Oregon and Patrick Leahy of Vermont, wrote to the FDA, "The regulatory uncertainty surrounding FDA's inaction has led to a proliferation of 'gluten free' standards and labels provided by 3rd party groups. . . . We ask that you provide us with an update on when FDA will promulgate a final rule, why FDA has taken so long to issue this rule, and if there are any legal or regulatory hurdles that have prevented the timely implementation of this rule."⁴⁶ Rather than answering Wyden and Leahy directly, Taylor announced that the agency had reopened the comment period on the rule it had proposed four years earlier. "Before finalizing our gluten-free definition," he stated, "we want up-to-date input from affected consumers, the food industry, and others to help assure [sic] that the label strikes the right balance. We must take into account the need to protect individuals with celiac disease from adverse health consequences while ensuring that food manufacturers can meet the needs of consumers by producing a wide variety of gluten-free foods."⁴⁷

"Gluten and the FDA: What's Taking So Long?" asked Andrea, a woman with celiac, in October 2011. "Right now," she continued, "pretty much anybody can stick a 'gluten-free' label on their packaging without proving it" (October 3, 2011). The *New York Times* editorial board posed the same question in August 2013, when the FDA finalized the rule it had first proposed six year earlier. The board wrote that it was "not clear why it has taken the food agency almost seven years to come up with a limit of 20 parts of gluten per million in products sold as 'gluten free,' a level similar to what is required in Canada and the European Union."⁴⁸

The most compelling answer may be that this was business as usual. A 2022 *Politico* investigation of the Center for Food Safety and Applied Nutrition, the FDA division responsible for food issues, provided numerous examples of unacceptable delay. A 2011 food safety reform act had instructed the agency to institute safety standards for agricultural water to prevent deadly foodborne illness outbreaks. Ten years later the FDA issued a proposed rule, but by 2022 still had not finalized or implemented it. Because the FDA had long argued that reducing sodium in food was a critical public health concern, the Institute of Medicine (a nonprofit group now known as the National Academy of Medicine) in 2010 urged the agency to establish mandatory sodium standards. Instead, it set voluntary standards; a decade later it still had failed to issue them. The FDA established a work group to study toxic elements in the food supply in 2017 but then ignored the group's suggestions. In response to pressure from health organizations and Congress, the agency announced that it would set standards for the presence of heavy metal in some baby foods. The deadline the agency gave itself, however, was several years away.[49] Viewed in the light of those incidents, the FDA's long delay in issuing a final rule about gluten may not have been unusual.

According to the report, gross underfunding partly explains the center's failure to act quickly. In addition, the report noted that the center suffers "from a deep-seated culture of avoiding hard decisions and a near-paralyzing fear of picking serious fights with the food industry."[50] It is difficult to ascertain the industry's attitude toward standardizing the definition of "gluten free." According to the *Federal Register*, some food companies indicated that they wanted a clear definition as a way of leveling the playing field and promoting fair competition "because all manufacturers would have to adhere to the same requirements if they label their products 'gluten free.'"[51] But we have seen that food companies had opposed including gluten in FALCPA and that many wanted a less demanding standard than the one the FDA proposed. The food industry has many ways to influence government decisions, especially when government officials previously have worked for those companies.[52] Although Michael Taylor's long career in industry did not include stints with food manufacturers, he may well have been more hospitable to their demands than to those of patient organizations. Celiac disease advocates could not possibly offer a counterweight to whatever pressure the industry decided to exert.

Enforcing the Ruling

Announcing that food companies had until August 5, 2014, to bring their gluten-free products into compliance with the new standard, Taylor asserted that the deadline should not be a problem because many companies already abided by the new rule. Moreover, they had "a huge incentive to comply.... They want people to be confident."[53] Two studies offered confirmation. Both reported that even before the ruling went into effect, the level of gluten in the vast majority of products labeled gluten free was less than twenty ppm.[54]

Mindful of FDA's long delay in promulgating the standards, however, some celiac advocates were not convinced that the battle was over. Tricia Thompson, the founder of the Gluten Free Watchdog (GFWD), launched a campaign to pressure the FDA to enforce its ruling. A registered dietician, Thompson is the author of both popular and scientific publications, including articles in the *New England Journal of Medicine*, the *Journal of the Academy of Nutrition and Dietetics*, and the *Journal of Human Nutrition and Dietetics*. She has contributed to the Academy of Dietetics' *Nutrition Care Manual* and is a working group member of the Academy's Evidence Analysis Library project on celiac disease. In July 2014, shortly before the ruling took effect, she posted an "Action Alert" on the GFWD website, encouraging the entire community to take responsibility for policing mislabeled food. She had heard from a former FDA consumer-safety officer that the agency would act only after receiving more than one complaint. "*As a community,*" Thompson wrote, "*we must make sure that the FDA receives as many complaints as possible for every product we believe is misbranded*" (emphasis in original). Misbranding, she continued, could occur in three main areas: "incomplete warning," "gluten content at or above 20 parts per million," and "use of ingredients not allowed." The last especially needed an explanation. In addition to establishing a standard, the FDA had announced that the products labeled gluten free could not contain any of the following ingredients—malt, malt syrup, and malt extract. (Thompson coined the term "facial misbranding" to describe products labeled gluten free that contain prohibited ingredients.) Other ingredients, including extracts of rye, extracts of barley, hydrolyzed wheat protein, and hydrolyzed barley protein, were likely to be excluded after the FDA announced plans for hydrolyzed and fermented products. (The FDA published the final rule on August 13, 2020, and it went into effect two months later.) Thompson emphasized that although the GFWD would contact the FDA directly, "THIS IS NOT ENOUGH. IF WE WANT FDA TO ACT AND ACT QUICKLY WE ALL MUST MAKE OUR VOICES HEARD AS LOUDLY AS POSSIBLE."[55]

In August 2017 Thompson and a colleague filed a citizens' petition to the FDA listing several products containing prohibited ingredients that remained in stores. The petition also requested the establishment of protocols to improve surveillance, investigation, and enforcement of misbranded items.[56] The reply from the FDA arrived in February 2018: "We have not reached a decision on your petition within the first 180 days due to competing priorities. However, be advised that your petition is currently under active evaluation by our staff."[57] The headline of Thompson's February 2020 post was, "Enough Is Enough with Gluten-Free Misbranding: Contact FDA Today." In the text, she implored members of her community to write to all personnel of the Health and Human Services and the FDA. Her own letter, which she included as a sample, read in part, "The lack of enforcement of the gluten-free labeling rule is putting at risk the health of the people with celiac disease. It also is emboldening manufacturers to openly disregard the codified rule. As FDA is well aware, it was a long journey over several years to finalize the gluten-free labeling rule. Many responsible gluten-free food manufacturers have taken the time and resources to ensure their labeling practices comply with the rule. But the journey is not complete. . . . We ask that FDA promptly turn its attention to the manufacturers who blatantly are not in compliance."[58] Thompson also appealed to her fellow dietitians to join the letter-writing campaign.[59]

By the following month, March 2020, Thompson was able to report some progress. The headline of her post credited the celiac community: "Four of eight products recalled: YOU are making a difference!" She understood that the onset of the pandemic that month had complicated everyone's life and made it more difficult for some to find time to write letters. Nevertheless, she hoped at least a few of her readers would remain active. "If you have the energy during this trying time," she wrote, "please continue to send emails."[60] In July Thompson wrote to the FDA, thanking it for recalling six products and insisting that it recall six others.[61]

In January 2021, Thompson had a new success to report. The FDA finally had recalled eight Chef Myron's sauces. "It is huge these recalls are happening," she wrote, before adding, "These recalls are a long time coming. Gluten Free Watchdog first reported Chef Myron's to the FDA in 2014. We last filed a complaint on August 18, 2020. Unfortunately, these sauces are sold to various food service outlets, including schools, hospitals, military, and restaurants."[62] The news on other fronts was less satisfactory. The GFWD also had complained to the FDA as early as 2014 that Dandy Blend, an instant herbal beverage, had ingredients that were not permitted; nevertheless, the product still remained on store shelves in February 2021.[63] In May 2022 Thompson wrote to Susan Mayne, director of FDA's Center for Food Safety and Applied Nutrition, demanding to know why the agency still had not taken action on any products labeled gluten free containing barley ingredients.[64] In September 2023, Thompson and two GFWD attorneys sent comments to the FDA about "several issues in the reporting and recall process that would benefit from heightened Agency attention." Those included "the perception that manufacturers' needs are being prioritized in recalls."[65] At the time this book went to press, Thompson was continuing her campaign to convince the FDA to implement its rules.

Conclusion

A central goal of healthcare advocates has been to transform the balance of power between physicians and patients by narrowing the gap between medical and lay knowledge. Although little had differentiated the ideas and practices of doctors from those of laypeople throughout the nineteenth century, physicians could claim unique competence by the early twentieth century. They alone had access to diagnostic tools, and they spoke a language few patients could comprehend. Since the 1970s, however, patients have been able to learn more about their diseases, therapies, and prognoses.[66] Because medicine plays a minor role in celiac care, celiacs need a different kind of knowledge. Beginning in the early 2000s they have demanded the right to make informed choices about the food labeled gluten free that they purchase and consume. After joining allergy groups in their struggle for passage of FALCPA, advocates spearheaded a campaign to force the FDA to clarify the term "gluten-free"; since then they have pressed the agency to implement its rule. The actions of profit-making food companies combined with the inaction of that agency have left people with celiac in a vulnerable position.

4

Patient Advocacy, Corporate Funding, and the Cheerios Debacle

The proliferation of health-advocacy organizations (HAOs) has directed attention to their conflicts of interest. HAOs are nonprofit groups that seek to raise awareness about a particular disease, increase research funding for it, and provide information and services to patients. Most rely heavily on financial donations from corporations. A 2017 study published in the *New England Journal of Medicine* reported that of the 104 HAOs reviewed, 83 percent received funds from pharmaceutical, medical-device, and biotechnology companies; 39 percent of the groups that disclosed the contributions received at least $1 million annually from industry.[1] In 2009 congressional investigators found that drug makers had contributed two-thirds of the donations to the National Alliance on Mental Illness between 2006 and 2008.[2] Critics focus not only on the high level of corporate funding but also on the failure of HAOs to reveal critical details.[3] "As highly trusted organizations," historian Sheila M. Rothman and colleagues write, "HAOs should disclose all corporate grants, including the purpose and the amount. Absent the disclosure, legislators, regulators, and the public cannot evaluate possible conflicts of interest or biases."[4]

Some researchers caution us against assuming that financial relationships between those groups and the pharmaceutical industry automatically result in cooptation. An Irish study found that those relationships take many forms and do not necessarily represent "corporate colonization."[5] Nevertheless, critics charge that industry funding has influenced some HAOs to support access to therapies that offer few benefits to patients and to endorse policies that do not serve members' interests.[6]

Although little research has examined financial relationships between the food industry and HAOs, members of the Food Allergy and Anaphylaxis Network have criticized the group's acceptance of donations from certain food companies.[7] Consumer and food activists have complained about the ties between the American Diabetes Association (ADA) and Cadbury-Schweppes, the largest confectioner in the world; for many years boxes of sugar-rich cookies displayed the ADA logo, proclaiming the company a "proud sponsor" of the association. Although the ADA established new guidelines for corporate sponsorship in 2008, some activists asserted that they were insufficient. "Maybe the American Diabetes Association should rename itself the American Junk Food Association," remarked Gary Ruskin, director of Commercial Alert, a consumer advocacy group. Other critics charged that the ADA's close ties with the pharmaceutical industry influenced the association to emphasize drug treatments in favor of lifestyle changes that could prevent disease.[8] Below I explore the extent to which industry funding may have encouraged celiac advocacy organizations to overstate the benefits of drug therapies and minimize criticisms of unhealthy food products (including some possibly containing unacceptable levels of gluten).

Celiac Disease Advocacy Groups

Five major celiac advocacy organizations provide essential services to the celiac community. The first was the Gluten Intolerant Group (GIG), founded in 1974. Its primary enterprise is administering the Gluten-Free Certification Organization (GFCO), a database for products tested to ensure that they have no more than ten ppm (parts per million) of gluten (half the FDA standard). Manufacturers who complete an eight-step process can place the GFCO mark on their products.[9] GIG also helps organize support groups, offers special programs for children, provides a validation program for staff in diverse institutions, and sends gluten-free food to those who are food insecure. In 2022, its revenue was $5.3 million.[10]

The National Celiac Association (NCA) was founded in 1977 as the Celiac Sprue Association. It provides education and support for people with celiac through various conferences, workshops, and both print and social media. It also has a gluten-testing program, which tries to ensure that gluten-free items contain five ppm or less of gluten (half the limit of the GIG program). The NCA is smaller than the other organizations, with a revenue of just $279,000 in 2020.[11]

Founded in California in 1990, the Celiac Disease Foundation (CDF) offers a broad array of programs and services in three main areas: advocacy, education, and medical research. Advocacy priorities include raising awareness of celiac disease among elected officials, strengthening gluten-free labeling regulations, including coverage of dietitians and nutritionists in Medicare and Medicaid, and increasing government funding for celiac research. Education programs serve both providers and the public; student ambassadors seek to increase celiac awareness among their peers. The foundation's iCureCeliac patient registry enables patients to determine whether they are eligible for different clinical trials. In addition, the organization funds research studies and holds both symposiums and seminars for researchers. The organization's revenue was $3.3 million in 2022.[12]

Beyond Celiac, founded in 2003 as the National Foundation for Celiac Awareness, defines its mission as "uniting with patients and partners to drive diagnosis, advance research, and accelerate the discovery of new treatments and a cure."[13] With a large patient database, the organization participates actively in patient recruitment for clinical trials. In addition, it awards research grants, hosts science summits, and presents original research. In 2022, its revenue was $3.3 million.[14]

The fifth organization is the Gluten Free Watchdog (GFWD), founded by Tricia Thompson in 2011. As noted in the last chapter, Thompson is a registered dietician who has written both popular and scientific publications. The primary mission of GFWD is to serve as an independent gluten testing organization. By 2019, the organization had tested more than seven hundred products. The results are reported on the organization's social media platforms. In addition, GFWD contacts both the manufacturer and the Food and Drug Administration (FDA) when foods making a gluten-free claim include ingredients that are not permitted in items labeled gluten free.[15] GFWD also engages in advocacy, especially with regard to the FDA.

Pharmaceutical Companies

Drug makers began to focus on celiac early in the twenty-first century, when studies about the prevalence of the disease appeared. Twenty-four therapies were in various stages of development by June 2022. The following month the trial for Larazotide, the drug that was farthest along, was discontinued, greatly disappointing the celiac community.[16] Nevertheless, researchers continue to invest considerable hope in the treatments that remain in the pipeline.[17] Two organizations, the Celiac Disease Foundation and Beyond Celiac, have close associations with the pharmaceutical industry; neither group, however, discloses whatever financial arrangements the partnerships include.

Here it is important to stress that developing a drug therapy is in celiacs' interest. As we will see in chapter 8, many feel excluded from the various social, religious, and family events that center on food. Even those who rigorously follow the prescribed diet worry about inadvertently ingesting enough gluten to harm the small intestine. Many advocates cite a 2014 study that found that people with celiac report a higher treatment burden than those with many other chronic conditions.[18] A 2022 study from the Celiac Disease Center at Columbia University found that 78 percent of the respondents had an interest in "non-dietary therapies" to enable them to broaden their diet, and 70 percent hoped such treatments would lessen the risk of cancer. When asked what side effects would make the medications unacceptable, they mentioned vomiting (80 percent) and weight gain (74 percent).[19]

Moreover, both Beyond Celiac and the Celiac Disease Foundation facilitate patient involvement in research, the goal of many health advocates. One of the achievements of AIDS activists in the 1980s and 1990s was what medical sociologist Steven Epstein calls "gaining a seat at the table," helping to influence the direction of HIV research.[20] In November 2021, Marilyn Geller, CEO of the Celiac Disease Foundation, wrote that she had just concluded a three-year term on the Advisory Panel on Patient Engagement of the Patient-Centered Outcomes Research Institute, a nonprofit institute created by the Affordable Care Act; part of its function is to enable patients and caregivers to contribute to research.[21] One of the services the foundation offers pharmaceutical companies is the opportunity to "solicit feedback and gather valuable insights from patients to improve your study feasibility, recruitment, and retention."[22] In May 2023 Geller wrote that the foundation had "engaged patients as key stakeholders in the research process by inviting them to participate in surveys, focus groups, webinars, workshops, conferences, and advisory boards—and each time they have answered the call to share their perspectives, preferences, and experience on various aspects of celiac disease research."[23]

Because drug therapies for celiac disease are still in development, the questions raised about the links between other HAOs and pharmaceutical companies are irrelevant here. We cannot ask, for example, whether celiac organizations promote policies that benefit drug makers more than patients. But we can ask whether the groups foster inflated expectations. The *Beyond Celiac Newsletter* of February 2023 displays a photograph of the CEO, Alice Bast, beneath a banner headline reading "Together for a cure!" The website also lists the "Barriers to a Cure for Celiac Disease." They include the following: "Celiac disease is poorly understood by the medical community; serious nature of the disease is underappreciated; lack of funding and strategic focus for research; limited support for early career scholars/researchers; too many people remain undiagnosed; assumption that the gluten-free diet is enough."[24] Those are all major impediments to celiac research. What is missing is any recognition that the drugs currently in development will serve merely as adjuncts to the gluten-free diet, not a cure for celiac. Only a vaccine, sometimes referred to as "the holy grail" of celiac research, would eradicate the disease, but it is much farther away than other potential therapies.[25]

The Celiac Disease Foundation also promises far more than is likely to be delivered, at least in the near future. I recently received an email message from the organization titled "We Can Cure Celiac Disease... If You Help." The message urges me to watch *Curing Celiac: A Short Story*, a film sponsored by the foundation. The film opens with several children playing soccer while a group of parents watch from the sidelines. When one mother opens a box containing an assortment of donuts, all the children but one run excitedly toward her and make their choices. The exception is a sad girl who lags behind. At home, the father comforts the girl by telling her about the ongoing research for celiac. The film explains why patients should join "iCureCeliac®," a public registry for celiac research.[26] To be sure, both Beyond Celiac and the Celiac Disease Foundation often refer to "treatments," as well as "a cure." The implication, however, is that the first leads automatically to the second. "Such is the power of the discourse of cure," writes Michael Bérubé, a literary critic and disability studies scholar, "it obliterates all nuance before and behind it."[27]

Finally, we might ask if the pharmaceutical companies that fund celiac organizations will expect a payback from them. When the drugs are in a later stage of development, will the organizations be expected to advocate for them in the regulatory process, minimize any possible side effects, justify costs that some might consider excessive, and argue for coverage by public and private insurance? The actions of other health-advocacy organizations suggest that these could become pertinent questions.[28]

Partnerships with the Food Industry

Alone among the five major celiac advocacy organizations, the Gluten Free Watchdog (GFWD) led by Tricia Thompson is funded entirely by subscriptions and accepts no manufacturers' advertisements or sponsorships. A headline on its website in 2017 underlined Thompson's disapproval of corporate funding: "When Sponsorship Dollars Muddy the Messaging for Products Sold to the Gluten-Free Community."[29]

The other four organizations have ties to gluten-free food manufacturers and solicit financial contributions from them.[30] Those organizations have demonstrated their independence from the food industry by calling for greater regulation. We saw that representatives of both the Celiac Disease Foundation and the Gluten Intolerance Group joined the American Celiac Task Force, established in 2003 to lobby Congress for passage of the Food Allergen Labeling and Consumer Protection Act (FALCPA), which many food companies vigorously opposed.[31] The Celiac Sprue Association (now the NCA) urged the Food and Drug Administration to set the standard for gluten in food labeled gluten-free far below the level demanded by the food industry. More recently, the major celiac associations have joined the campaign to pass the Food Labeling Modernization Act of 2023, an updated version of a bill introduced in 2018, which would fill a major gap in FALCPA for celiacs by requiring the disclosure of barley and rye in addition to wheat.[32]

Nevertheless, some commentators charge that the close ties between those organization and the food industry are a cause for concern. In what follows I focus on the Celiac Disease Foundation because its alliance with major food companies has received the most criticism. According to the 2023 annual report, "Corporate sponsorships account for approximately 22% of the Foundation's annual budget."[33] Although the foundation's website notes that the organization offers several levels of sponsorship ("Leadership," "Champion," "Major," "Premier," "Elite," and "Supporting"), it does not indicate what financial contribution is required for each. With the exception of Glutenostics, a company designing a mobile app to improve celiac diagnosis, all the corporate sponsors are food companies. General Mills (GM) is one of the six groups listed as "Leadership Sponsors." Three of the others are Nature Valley, Chex, and Cheerios, all of which are GM brands.[34] As we will see, the foundation has defended GM's Cheerios' gluten-free label, although many critics charge that the product is unsafe for people with celiac.

Sponsorship enables companies to simultaneously burnish their reputations and advance their marketing agendas. They can place a logo with the words "Celiac Disease Proud Sponsor" on their products. In addition, the company logo is displayed on celiac.org, the foundation's website, as well as on announcements of the foundation's various educational programs and fundraising events; the company is granted a preferred placement in the annual gluten-free exposition; and the company name appears in the annual report. Celiac.org provides familiar information about living with celiac disease: "The most cost-effective and healthy way to follow the gluten-free diet is to seek out these naturally gluten-free food groups, which include fruits, vegetables, meat and poultry, fish and seafood, dairy, beans, legumes, and nuts. . . . Many items that usually contain gluten have gluten-free alternatives that are widely available in most grocery stores. . . . It is very important to base your diet around fruits, vegetables, meats, and other healthy food groups."[35]

As already noted, medical professionals offer similar advice, encouraging celiacs to limit the amount of ultraprocessed foods they consume in favor of products that are naturally free of gluten. But publicizing this message widely is not in the interest of the food companies that fund the foundation, and their logos and advertisements drown it out. A 2023 study from the Celiac Disease Center at Columbia University of eighty celiacs found that their average level of consumption of ultraprocessed food was higher than experts recommend (though lower than among the general population).[36]

The entanglement of marketing and advocacy goals is perhaps clearest in the app "Eat! Gluten-Free," which can be downloaded from both the Apple App Store and the Google Play Store. The foundation describes the app this way: "You are eating gluten-free, either by doctor's orders or by choice, and you have questions:—What is safe to eat?—How can I safely prepare gluten-free food?—What tastes good?—What are the nutrition facts? Eat! Gluten-Free is the most trusted source for all of your gluten-free needs, built and managed by the Celiac Disease Foundation."[37] Companies are invited to pay to have their brands mentioned in the products list, featured in banner ads, and included in recipes. The first recipe, for example, is for almond butter apple granola wedges. The ingredients include one apple, two teaspoons of almond butter, and two–three tablespoons of Jessica's granola. The instructions are to "cut apples into wedges, drizzle almond butter on top of apples, sprinkle with Jessica's Granola." A banner at the top of the page reads, "Jessica's Natural Foods." Clicking on the link leads to a page about the company, which begins, "Here at Jessica's Natural Foods we are passionate about natural food. Our family reads a lot of labels when we are grocery shopping, and we are finicky about what we bring home. We only want the best all-natural, non-GMO and/or organic food for our family, so naturally these are the kinds of products we produce." The page contains information about contacting the company as well as a link to its website.[38]

Eat!Gluten-Free also includes various meal plans that provide "three meals and two snacks each day with easy to make recipes and 'Quick Fixes' for those on-the-go." The "7-Day Meal Plan" opens with an advertisement for Schär's gluten-free products, including a link to the online shop. The breakfast for day five consists of sausage egg muffins, which fits two cuisines, "Kid Friendly" and "Mother's Day." At the top of the recipe is the name "Jones Dairy Farm." A link connects to a page of information about that company, which begins, "Jones Dairy Farm is a seventh-generation family owned and operated business located in Fort Atkinson, Wisconsin. For more than 130 years Jones Dairy Farm has been making distinctive quality, clean label products starting with their signature All Natural breakfast sausage." The muffins' ingredients include a cup of Jones Dairy Farm Sausage.[39] Far from being a "trusted source," the app appears to function at least in part as a marketing tool.

Gluten-Free Cheerios

The Celiac Disease Foundation's statements about the gluten-free Cheerios first produced by General Mills (GM) in 2015 increased suspicion of the role of corporate finance in the organization. By that year

GM occupied a major place in the gluten-free market. Best known for Betty Crocker and Pillsbury as well as Cheerios, the company is one of the four corporations that control 86 percent of the $8.6 billion breakfast cereal market.[40] A cereal manufacturer might seem to be an unlikely entity to align itself with the gluten-free craze. Although health-conscious entrepreneurs introduced cold cereal in the 1860s, the major companies more recently have become notorious for their contribution to the children's obesity epidemic. Between 1980 and 2018, the proportion of children who were either overweight or obese increased from 15 percent to 35 percent; those who were Black, Hispanic, or came from families that were socioeconomically disadvantaged had the highest levels.[41] In 2005 the Institute of Medicine confirmed what had long been known, that "food and beverage marketing practices geared to children and youth are out of balance with recommended healthful diets and contribute to an environment that puts their health at risk."[42] A 2009 study from the Rudd Center for Food Policy and Obesity at Yale University reported that large cereal companies targeted children with advertisements for products with poor nutritional value and high sugar content. Children's cereals contained 85 percent more sugar, 65 percent less fiber, and 60 percent more sodium than adult cereals. General Mills was the outlier, responsible for 60 percent of all cereal advertisements targeting children.[43] A follow-up study in 2012 reported that cereal companies had improved the nutritional quality of their products but continued to advertise the least healthy ones to children. General Mills again stood out, this time as the only company to increase cereal advertisements targeting children and youth of all ages.[44]

But health claims increase sales. Warren J. Belasco demonstrates that the food industry responded to the countercultural cuisine of the 1960s by reformulating and repackaging some products as organic or natural.[45] Taking the lead in that endeavor, cereal manufacturers soon began introducing items labeled "100 percent natural." In the 1980s and 1990s, the companies launched low-fat alternatives to familiar products.[46] A drop in cereal consumption at the turn of the twenty-first century provided a new incentive to refashion certain brands and advertise them as healthier. Many people who previously had viewed cold cereal as the most convenient way to start the day now preferred to grab a piece of fruit or a breakfast bar at a fast-food counter. Many of those who still had breakfast at home prepared oatmeal, cooked eggs, or toasted frozen waffles, French toast, and pancakes instead of pouring a bowl of cereal.[47] The proportion of Americans eating cereal for the morning meal slipped from 38 percent in 1996 to 29 percent by 2014.[48] Appealing to health-minded consumers became an attractive way to try to recoup the loss.

For many years, GM had won praise for its policies and practices regarding food allergies. Unlike most other food companies, it provided an extensive list of ingredients on package labels, educated employees about food allergies, kept a detailed database about the presence of allergens in different products, and readily answered customers who called to ask about specific items.[49] Reviews of the company's record in the gluten-free market, however, were far less positive. The company's first foray into that market was Gluten-Free Rice Chex, launched in 2008. Jim Murphy, president of the company's cereal division, soon boasted that Chex, long a "pretty sleepy" brand, had been given "a real jolt."[50] Betty Crocker introduced gluten-free brownies, cookies, desserts, and cake mixes in 2009 and a pancake mix in 2010. By 2011, the company also had placed gluten-free labels on hundreds of items that naturally contained no gluten.[51] That year, GM launched Gluten Freely, an online site for gluten-free products, most of which were still local and thus not widely available. GlutenFreely delivered to customers' doors items from Udi's in Colorado, Dr. Schärs in Italy, Pamela's in California, and Barkat in England. The site had more than 110,000 users within the first six months. It closed in 2013, by which time many more retailers carried gluten-free products.[52] Acquisitions also helped General Mills become a major player in the gluten-free market. In 2000 GM had enlarged its wellness profile by purchasing Small Planet Foods, a leading producer of organic and natural food.[53] In 2012, Small Planet Foods bought Food Should Taste Good, a gluten-free snack food business.[54]

Early in 2015, GM announced that it would take a bigger risk, offering gluten-free versions of Cheerios, its iconic brand. First introduced in 1941 as Cheeri Oats, the cereal was renamed in 1945. New flavors began to appear in 1976.[55] The five Cheerios varieties GM planned to reformulate as gluten free included Original, Honey Nut, Apple Cinnamon, Frosted, and Multi-Grain; together they represented 88 percent of all cereals GM offered.[56] Because the main ingredient of Cheerios is oats, refashioning the different varieties was a far more complicated process than it had been with Chex, made with rice. Although oats are naturally free of gluten, they are often contaminated in the production process. To avoid cross-contamination, people with celiac often are advised to consume only those grown under a "purity protocol" ensuring that they are and remain gluten free. The suppliers release their testing protocols and provide extensive information about the process used to avoid contamination.[57] GM, however, decided to save money by mechanically cleaning oats at the back end of production rather than using only the more expensive oats specially grown to be gluten free. Although that decision required the company to build a special facility to clean and sort the oats, it was less expensive than buying purity oats.

By 2015, consumers had reason to be wary of GM's marketing promises about Cheerios. In September 2007 the front of yellow Cheerios boxes had displayed a heart with this assertion printed over it: "You can lower your cholesterol 4% in 6 weeks." The inscription on the back of the box read, "Cheerios is the only leading cold cereal clinically proven to lower cholesterol. A clinical study showed that eating 1 and ½ cup servings daily of Cheerios cereal reduced cholesterol when eaten as part of a diet low in saturated fat and cholesterol."[58] In May 2009, the FDA sent GM a warning letter about its misleading claims.[59] A few months later a woman in California filed a class-action lawsuit alleging that General Mills had made false assertions about the effect of Cheerios on cholesterol and heart disease.[60] In 2014 GM announced that it would make a GMO-free version of Cheerios, although it previously had stated that the cereal never had been GMO. Marion Nestle commented snidely that the company now "will take extra trouble—and, no doubt, charge more—to make sure the GMO and non-GMO sugars and corn don't mix."[61]

Those incidents help to explain why some members of the gluten-free community responded to GM's announcement of gluten-free Cheerios with skepticism. One was a blogger who had been diagnosed with celiac and called himself "Gluten Dude." By that time he had earned a reputation for his confrontational stance toward the food industry. Three years earlier he had written that he had lost weight, gained energy, and felt healthier when he began to eat only whole foods that were naturally gluten free. He urged his readers to follow his example: "A large majority of the gluten-free food is absolute garbage. And many (not all) of the gluten-free food manufacturers are more than happy to feed us this crap because they know the emotional attachment people have with eating. And they know the intense fear celiacs have of losing their lifestyle as they know it. And they know the enormous profit they can make off of us."[62]

When Gluten Dude heard about the launch of GM's Cheerios early in March 2015, he asked the question that would bedevil many critics for years: "How will [the Cheerios] be gluten-free when their main ingredient is oats and as we all know, unless you use certified gluten-free oats, the risk of cross contamination is extremely high?" Gluten Dude also doubted the company's commitment to transparency: "GM says they are using a proprietary method that they have been working on for years that removes all traces of wheat, barley, and rye from their cereal. Now the word 'proprietary' usually sets off some alarm bells in my head." He soon had a way to address his concerns. The company invited him to attend what it called "a gluten-free forum, an intimate group of gluten-free leaders meeting March 25–26 at the General Mills headquarters in Minneapolis." Despite his hesitancy, Gluten Dude decided to go. "Will I eat the Cheerios while there?" he asked rhetorically. "Not until I learn ALL about their methods."[63]

Another participant at the forum, Jennifer North, vice president of the National Foundation for Celiac Awareness, wrote on her return, "General Mills and the Cheerios team have their work cut out for them as they flush and clean not only the entire mill, but also their huge grain elevators and transportation fleet of trucks and railcars. What an undertaking! ... Cheerios labeled gluten-free will begin appearing this summer with full distribution around September. It may take some stores up to a year to run through their current stock so **be careful to look for the gluten-free label**" (emphasis in original).[64] Marilyn Geller, the CEO of the Celiac Disease Foundation, later recalled that she had "listened as General Mills outlined the millions of dollars it had invested in its sourcing, manufacturing, packaging, and shipping processes to assure that, going forward, Cheerios were indeed gluten free."[65] Gluten Dude, however, remained dubious. He had quickly discovered that he fit uneasily into the group of advocates at the forum. On his return, he noted that he had been the only one not invited to be interviewed by video. "I don't belong at GM helping them to promote their products," he concluded. When asked specifically whether celiacs should trust gluten-free Cheerios, he equivocated, "While I'm confident in the process, until the final product comes out and is tested by a third party (aka Gluten Free Watchdog), I will not recommend for or against trying them. Time will tell."[66] In June 2015, Tricia Thompson, the founder and head of the Gluten Free Watchdog, released her decision. She did "**not support the use of regular oats that are cleaned at the 'end' of production via mechanical and/or optical sorting to be 'gluten-free'**" (emphasis in original).[67]

Events in July suggested that her caution was warranted. Soon after the first shipments of Cheerios arrived in supermarkets, consumers began to complain that they had become ill. GFWD posted numerous letters, many of which followed the same format. The writers expressed their delight in learning that they could eat their favorite cereal again and their deep disappointment upon discovering it could not be trusted. "My husband brought Gluten Free Honey Nut Cheerios home from the grocery store yesterday," Ellen wrote. "I was so thrilled to see they were gluten free. I had about a cup of the new Cheerios with milk for breakfast and boy did I get sick! I knew they weren't gluten free. ... Shame on General Mills!" The mother of two children with celiac wrote that she was "excited to find the GF labeled Cheerios on the shelf and thus purchased a box for my children. . . . I started seeing differences in their behavior after just two days of eating the cereal. I have now gone back and read all these blog posts about Cheerios and I'm kicking myself for getting so excited about their offer of a new 'gluten free' product and overriding my abundance of caution. I will not be buying any more." Thompson urged writers to contact General Mills and the FDA's MedWatch.[68]

In a post titled "Pissing in the Gluten-Free Cheerios," Debi Smith, a blogger, noted that the controversy surrounding gluten-free Cheerios had caused "a divide. On one side are people who are encouraging people to eat them and eating it themselves. On the other side are people like me who are staying far away from them and will never encourage anyone with any type of issue with gluten to eat them." Because "more and more stories of people in the gluten free community kept pouring in," Smith had started a petition on Change.org. "The only thing that you have to be to sign this petition," she wrote, "is a human being who believes Celiac/gluten-sensitive people should be able to enjoy labeled gluten-free foods safely."[69] By September 29, the petition had garnered 2,100 signatures; 169 were from people who stated that they had become sick after eating gluten-free Cheerios.[70]

In the middle of August, Thompson reiterated her conclusion: "Based on the totality of information provided to GFWD, it is our position at this time that individuals with celiac disease should not eat gluten-free Cheerios. Before Gluten Free Watchdog can feel comfortable with this product, General Mills must take steps to ensure that Cheerios is not contaminated with barley (apparently the most problematic grain when it comes to mechanically 'cleaning' oats)."[71] GM's testing method was an especially serious problem. The FDA relied on companies to test their own product and intervened only after receiving complaints. GM decided to test several lots to find the mean rather than testing each box individually. Thompson pointed out that the presence of gluten in one box might be diluted by another.

Thompson also posted the contradictory statements from GM in response to questions she had posed through email. The company declared both that "it is not accurate to say that General Mills is not interested in purchasing pure oats for gluten free Cheerios and other products" and that "at this time you should not have any expectation that Cheerios will be moving to a purity protocol."[72] Other celiac community leaders who pressed GM for more information about Cheerios similarly met obfuscation. Gluten Dude wrote to his contact at GM at the end of September, "I know you guys have been getting pretty slammed. And I know that many in the celiac community have gotten quite sick from eating Cheerios. It seems obvious to me that your 'mean' testing is not sufficient. Any thoughts on what you are going to do to improve the situation?" The response came not from his contact but rather from the brand media relations manager, who asserted that the problem lay with the sufferers, not with the product they consumed: "Cheerios are safe—and they are gluten free. But celiac disease is a complex condition, and dietary changes for people with celiac disease often require the assistance of a trained physician. Dietary restrictions are individual and unique. Before introducing new foods into the diet, even gluten free oat products, experts routinely recommend that people with celiac disease or gluten sensitivity consult first with their treating physician."[73] Alice Bast, CEO of the National Foundation for Celiac Awareness (NFCA, later Beyond Celiac), explained what kind of communication could inspire trust. Her group had "been in ongoing dialogue with General Mills to provide clarity on the validation of its testing methods. When working with gluten-free food manufacturers, NFCA expects both transparency and the utmost caution when making a gluten-free claim. . . . I'm left to wonder why it feels like you need a Ph.D. to navigate the gluten-free testing methods and protocols for producing food that is really gluten free."[74]

Although Erin Smith, a social media influencer, had conducted extensive research before speaking by phone to GM "marketing representatives," she, too, remained frustrated. "I asked my readers and Facebook fans to share their concerns and comments with me," she wrote. "I watched all their videos and read the FAQ pages to educate myself about the gluten-free Cheerios process." Like many others, she deferred to Tricia Thompson, reading "all the scientific reports on Gluten Free Watchdog." Smith also ensured that everything else she read "was recent," rather than "driven by the blogger promotional trip to General Mills" the previous spring. "I was prepared," she stressed. Nevertheless, she received little satisfaction: "I got off the call feeling like the celiac community isn't safe eating these new Cheerios despite the years of research and development. I really do not think General Mills is quite there yet with a truly gluten-free product and that the complaints of people getting sick need to be taken very seriously."[75]

Nevertheless, General Mills had reason to be pleased with the Cheerios rollout. On September 22, *Fortune* reported that the company already was seeing signs that its "big bet" was "paying off." GM's cereal sales had risen 6 percent in the previous quarter.[76] *Business Insider* quoted a company spokesperson who said that gluten-free Cheerios was destined to be "one of the largest merchandising events in our cereal business history."[77]

But then, on October 5, General Mills announced that it had recalled 1.8 million boxes of gluten-free Yellow Box Cheerios and Honey Nut Cheerios that had been contaminated.[78] "Our Lodi [California] production facility lost rail service for a time and our gluten-free oat flour was being off-loaded from rail cars to trucks for delivery to our facility on the dates in question," Jim Murphy explained. "In an isolated incident involving purely human error, wheat flour was inadvertently introduced into our gluten-free oat flour system at Lodi." Murphy added that he was "embarrassed and truly sorry" for the problem.[79]

Several advocates now redoubled their criticism of General Mills and Cheerios. "I am livid by this whole situation," Erin Smith wrote. "First and foremost, General Mills put wheat flour into a product that was supposed to be gluten-free. Period. **WHEAT IS NOT GLUTEN-FREE.** This is Gluten and celiac disease 101. How did 'human error' allow for enough wheat flour to be introduced into the production process to affect 1.8 million boxes of Cheerios? Did not one single person notice trucks with wheat entering this facility?"[80] Shirley Braden wrote on her blog *Glutenfreeeasily.com*, "**Stop eating gluten-free Cheerios. I reiterate. Do not eat General Mills 'gluten-free' Cheerios**. . . . I'm not simply talking about abstaining from eating the 'gluten-free' Cheerios that were included in the recall of October 8, 2016. . . . I'm telling you to abstain from **all** 'gluten-free' Cheerios. DO NOT EAT ANY 'GLUTEN-FREE' CHEERIOS. Period."[81] The founder of *Alivewithoutgluten.com* wrote, "I rarely post something quickly without taking at least a day or two to make sure I'm not overly angry, happy, or any other emotion that could be affecting how rational I'm being about the matter. I'm deciding to make an exception. I've been putting a lot of thought into all of the controversy surrounding Cheerios for the last several months, and I'll admit that I could not stop being angry or frustrated this whole time. I'm now at my tipping point."[82]

Tricia Thompson and Gluten Dude focused on GM's concealment and duplicity. Two days after the announcement, Thompson wrote an open letter to the company. The recall "and subsequent explanation of how these products made it to market has raised many questions. One of the biggest concerns is the apparent discrepancy between what you told the community about your testing protocols and what you were actually doing." She noted that two months earlier GM had sent Gluten Dude as well as other members of the community an assurance that "the finished product [is] tested for safety a final time." Why, then, Thompson asked, were the recalled boxes not tested a final time?[83] Gluten Dude also accused GM of secrecy, questioning why General Mills waited until October to reveal an incident that had occurred in July. "Look," he wrote, "do I think the folks at GM are evil people who are intentionally poisoning us for profit? No I don't. But damn. Transparency goes such a long way, especially within our community. Instead of denying for months that your product was causing our community harm, don't you wish you kept the lines of communication open just a bit more?" He concluded,

"So disgusted. So disappointed. So tired of needing to write these kind of posts."

The Celiac Disease Foundation immediately alerted its members to the recall. In addition, it posted several irate letters on its Facebook page. "My son is 4 and has celiac," one parent wrote. "His allergy is very serious. He has ate [sic] cheerios for the last couple of weeks. He has been sick off and on for 2 weeks. We have tried to think of anything that could be causing it and blamed it on the school. Last night he got really sick with a severe allergic reaction and spent the night in the ER and all day today at his pediatrician's office. He is miserable. Came home and checked the box we have open right now and sure enough, it's the same code." The letter concluded, "My heart is broken as I watch our little guy suffer."[84]

But the foundation's tone differed from that of several other advocates. Noting that GM had been its "partner for many years," Marilyn Geller, the CEO, wrote, "We fully understand and appreciate that it is **our** responsibility to do everything in our power to hold General Mills accountable to the celiac disease and gluten sensitive communities. . . . In our meeting with General Mills yesterday, we were apprised of the new oat flour handling protocols and testing procedures for all finished products that have been implemented since the recall to assure that Cheerios labeled gluten-free meet the FDA standard. We expect General Mills to implement these new controls fully and continuously to earn back our community's trust." Geller also stressed that the recalls had been "voluntary," a claim GM often made.[85]

Although sales briefly dipped after the recall, the brand's overall trend continued upward. On December 21, 2015, CEO Ken Powell stated that the company's cereal sales had fallen 5 percent in the previous quarter, but the gluten-free Cheerios varieties had grown 3–4 percent. "The launch of gluten-free Cheerios is an important component of our cereal growth plan," he remarked, "and we're encouraged by the results."[86] Eighteen months later CEO Jeffrey Harmening told investors that GM had more than eight hundred gluten-free products across different brands. "We'll leverage our gluten-free news," he promised, because it demonstrates that the company promotes "wellness," a strategy that helps to stem the decline in cereal sales. A GM spokesperson told a reporter that the company "is confident our Cheerios and Lucky Charms cereals that are labeled 'gluten-free' meet the gluten free standard set by the FDA." Moreover, all cereals are tested "throughout production to ensure they meet and exceed the FDA standard. This includes testing finished products on every date of production at each of our production facilities, as well as testing our oat supply and our oat flour."[87]

Such avowals failed to convince everyone, especially as reports of sickness continued to pour in. In response to news that General Mills was introducing gluten-free Cheerios in Canada in July 2016, the Canadian Celiac Association issued a statement that although "some boxes of cereal in the market may be safe for people with celiac disease," others "contain significant gluten contamination that has not been detected using current testing protocols." As a result, "people with celiac disease or gluten sensitivity should not consume Cheerios products in spite of the gluten-free claim." In October 2017 the association announced that the Canadian Food Inspection Agency had announced that the words "gluten free" would be removed from all Cheerios sold in Canada by January 1, 2018.[88] Jocelyn Silvester, a Boston Children's Hospital physician, commented in 2017, "We recommend that patients with celiac disease avoid products made with mechanically-optically separated oats as it is unclear whether any given product is safe and there is no reliable tool to find out."[89]

The Celiac Disease Foundation, however, must have received the assurances it sought. After the Canadian Celiac Association recommended that people with celiac not consume gluten-free Cheerios in 2016, the foundation wrote, "Our Medical Advisory Board has no evidence that General Mills gluten-free cereals are not safe for celiac consumption. General Mills is a proud sponsor of Celiac Disease Foundation, and they understand the importance of safe gluten-free food to our community."[90] Continuing complaints of sickness also failed to alter the foundation's stance.[91]

Gluten Dude accused the foundation of catering to GM's interests. Why, he asked in July 2017, was the Celiac Disease Foundation (CDF) logo "on EVERY SINGLE BOX of Gluten-Free Cheerios? You know and I know what the an$wer i$. Becau$e it'$ alway$ the an$wer."[92] His followers underlined that point. "I am disappointed in General Mills for there [sic] careless and greedy decisions," one woman wrote, "but I'm beyond angered at CDF which has betrayed the trust of the very people it was founded to serve! Unforgivable!" Another woman commented that because she had been diagnosed many years earlier, she knew which brands she could trust. But if she were newly diagnosed or a parent who had just been told her child had celiac, the CDF seal of approval on the cereal boxes would reassure her that the cereal was safe to eat. "That's unconscionable. The CDF have no credibility. If they can't fund their programs any other way, then they shouldn't exist."[93]

In the same blog, Gluten Dude noted that he had written to the foundation requesting that it remove its logo from all Cheerios boxes "because they have NOT been proven to be safe for the celiac community." He added, "I know GM is one of your biggest sponsors, but it really should be community first."[94] The foundation response reiterated GM's argument that people who became sick from Cheerios must have a special intolerance to oats: "Since the voluntary recall of October of 2015, CDF has received no information from the FDA that Cheerios products pose a risk to people with celiac disease who can tolerate oats. Until such time that General Mills no longer wishes to support the celiac community, their gluten-free products will continue to bear the Celiac Disease Foundation logo."[95] We have seen that FDA enforcement is extremely lax; the organization thus could rest assured that a notification about Cheerios from the FDA was unlikely to arrive at any point in the near future.

The Cheerios debacle helps to explain why many celiac advocates erupted in fury in February 2020 when General Mills proposed developing a "gluten friendly" line, including biscuit mix, brownie mix, frozen biscuit dough, and frozen baked brownies. After a few restaurants were sued by people who claimed that they became ill after eating food labeled gluten free in restaurants, some promoted their menus as "gluten friendly" rather than "gluten free" to avoid possible liability.[96] General Mills now defined "gluten friendly" as "items manufactured without gluten-containing ingredients. General Mills does not claim these items meet FDA requirements for 'gluten-free' because of the possibility for cross contamination with gluten, including due to shared cooking and prep areas in kitchens."[97]

The response was immediate. The day after GM's announcement, one blogger wrote on Twitter, "Hey @General Mills, is this like your Cheerios? Maybe they should be changed to gluten-friendly too, since they still make people sick. You're doing it wrong . . . fix it. Your products are endangering the Celiac Community."[98] Tricia Thompson also posted a message that day: "@General Mills. Appalling. Gluten-friendly Pillsbury Biscuit Dough? Way to take a term that we're hoping to get rid of & escalate it. Gluten friendly has no meaning. This is a lazy attempt to sell products instead of ensuring safety for folks w/CD. Not good."[99] Thompson invited readers to send her comments, which she would compile and send to GM. Over and over readers charged GM with duplicity. One man, for example, commented, "'Gluten Friendly' is a very confusing term, and one that people in the food service industry will easily mistake for gluten free. Shortening Gluten Friendly to GF is misleading and will no doubt cause people with celiac disease to get glutened, making them sick. A note to General Mills: People with celiac disease must take our gluten free seriously. If you want us to be your customers, you must do the same. Be honest in your labeling so we can make educated decisions."[100] It is likely that the outcry from the celiac community had at least some impact because there is no evidence that General Mills ever produced a gluten-friendly line.

Criticism of GM's gluten-free Cheerios, however, has had little effect on the company. In March 2021, GFWD issued its "updated position statement on Cheerios." The "bottom line" was that "**Gluten Free Watchdog cannot in good conscience recommend gluten-free**

Cheerios."¹⁰¹ Two years later Tricia Thompson wrote that in the past two years she had found high levels of gluten in many of the oat products she tested. One possibility, she explained, was that the drought had drastically reduced the availability of purity-protocol oats. In April 2023 she announced, "Gluten Free Watchdog cannot recommend any brand of gluten-free oats. This includes products that are certified gluten-free or made using purity protocol oats."¹⁰²

This issue continues to divide the celiac community. Jenny Levine Finke's blog *Good for You Gluten Free* deplored GFWD's "extreme" position: "One can only assume that Thompson knows how overly-restrictive eating can take its toll on the gluten-free community. Hypervigilance can lead to eating disorders, mental and emotional anguish, food fear, anxiety, and disordered eating. . . . *Some* brands offer safe products. Painting the entire gluten-free oat industry with a single brush is not my style."¹⁰³ In November, the GFWD slightly modified its stance. The organization stated that although it still could not recommend any particular brand of gluten-free oats, people should make their own choices about whether or not to eat them.¹⁰⁴

Conclusion

Those who imply that a drug therapy will cure celiac disease follow a familiar script. As the sociologist Arthur W. Frank argues, we expect stories of illness to advance along a single plot line: "Yesterday I was healthy, today I'm sick, but tomorrow I'll be healthy again."¹⁰⁵ Advertisements for hospitals and pharmaceuticals display people radiantly smiling because they have been restored to health. And, of course, we all hope for a full recovery whenever we are ill. But celiacs who contribute financially to the research enterprise or participate in clinical trials expecting that a pill will eradicate the disease are likely to meet disappointment.

Most celiac advocacy organizations position the food industry as an ally in the fight for people with celiac, pointing to the organizations' many endeavors that could not exist without financial contributions from major manufacturers. That argument has considerable merit. The groups provide a number of programs and services that advance the interests of celiacs and enrich their lives; many undoubtedly rely on corporate funding. The issue is whether advocacy organizations remain beholden to their food-industry sponsors, even to the extent of ignoring complaints about products that some experts consider unsafe for celiacs. The controversy that arose in response to GM's production of gluten-free Cheerios demonstrates that that is a serious concern. Critics charged that the company concealed the process it used to sort the oats, relied on a testing protocol that could hide the presence of gluten, and provided contradictory statements in response to requests for further information. Those arguments have no place on the Celiac Disease Foundation's website.

5

"You're Not Crazy"

Getting—or Not Getting—a Diagnosis

"The delivery of health care has proceeded for decades with a blind spot," declared the National Academies of Sciences, Engineering, and Medicine in 2015. "Diagnosis errors—inaccurate or delayed diagnoses—persist throughout all settings of care and continue to harm an unacceptable number of patients."[1] Celiac disease represents an extreme example. Despite the efforts of advocacy groups, celiac disease centers, and pharmaceutical companies to increase celiac awareness, many people never learn they have the disease. Many others wait for the correct diagnosis for years. Members of both groups endure unnecessary suffering and remain at high risk of the serious conditions associated with untreated celiac, including osteoporosis and some forms of cancer.

Celiac diagnosis relies on serological tests, followed by an intestinal biopsy to confirm positive results. Because serological testing is now extremely accurate, researchers increasingly advocate avoiding the biopsy, especially for children. Current guidelines recommend testing for all first-degree relatives of people with celiac but not universal testing.[2]

A 2019 Mayo Clinic study reported that as many as half of all adults with celiac had not been diagnosed.[3] Researchers explain that finding by noting that doctors continue to be unaware that celiac disease is widespread, that the symptoms, especially among adults, are very varied, and that some patients are asymptomatic.[4] "This has been a very trying year for me," Terry wrote on the celiac.com forum. The previous year "a blood lab was done that showed me as celiac positive." Because she had no gastrointestinal symptoms, however, she "was told it was a false positive and to go about my life, unless symptoms showed" (November 29, 2016).

In a country without universal health care, lack of access to medical care also contributes to underdiagnosis. A college student explained on the forum that she had not received a biopsy after her positive blood test because she could not afford insurance coverage. Claire had managed to scrape together the money for an intestinal biopsy: "They did the blood work first, which is where they found I did have the antibodies, and then they told me I would need to follow up with an endoscopy. That was a lot of money, especially without insurance, and it took some time but I got there" (January 2, 2017). Violet had insurance but could obtain neither a blood test nor a biopsy. She wrote that although she had several celiac symptoms, "my insurance won't pay for [the tests] since I am not anemic and have no family history of celiac" (July 26, 2017). Members of racially marginalized groups are especially likely to lack insurance plans that would cover celiac tests. They also are less likely to be diagnosed because physicians and researchers have long assumed that the disorder primarily affects European whites.[5]

Another group of people do not appear in medical statistics because they have decided to dispense with standard tests and diagnose themselves. A major deterrent is the "gluten challenge"—eating substantial amounts of gluten for several weeks before receiving either a blood test or an endoscopy. One blogger abandoned the challenge after two and a half weeks because she "was so incredibly ill. . . . The lethargy, bloating, brain fog, irritability, nausea, headaches, joint pain, and everything else was just too much to bear."[6] Another wrote,

> It has been 7 years since I stopped eating/drinking gluten, and every time I am exposed to it—whether it be an accidental ingestion or cross-contamination—I fall extremely ill. . . . There is no question in my mind that I need to avoid gluten. The test to confirm celiac status would require me to begin ingesting it again for several weeks. . . . I read stories in forums and [Facebook] groups all the time of individuals putting themselves

through that hell just to get a doctor to confirm what they already know: that they shouldn't be ingesting gluten. These people often end up in the hospital because of their reactions, suffering greatly. No thank you.[7]

As this quotation indicates, people who are not convinced that doctors have anything to offer are especially likely to rely on self-diagnosis. One celiac-support-group member told two sociologists why he decided to forgo medical testing. After a friend suggested that celiac might be the cause of his fatigue and gastrointestinal problems, "I did a bit of reading on the internet and the symptoms kept ringing true to my situation. So I went on an informal [gluten-free diet], and after a few days I started feeling better. . . . But I thought, well maybe it's just my imagination. . . . So I went back to eating gluten again and after a couple days I was really sick. . . . so then I said, well maybe there is something to this! . . . It doesn't matter whether I get an official diagnosis or not if I feel lousy when I eat the stuff! What's the point going through all that agony and ending up at the same place?" Another sufferer simply said, "You don't need a prescription to go gluten free."[8]

The designation in 2008 of non-celiac gluten sensitivity (NCGS, also known as gluten sensitivity) as a distinct disorder strengthened the belief among some individuals that self-diagnosis is adequate. NCGS is basically a disease of elimination, meaning that other disorders have been ruled out and patients feel better after removing gluten from their diet. Because NCGS does not damage the small intestine, it is considered less serious than celiac; as a result, patients can be somewhat more lax in adhering to a gluten-free diet.[9] Because the treatment for celiac and NCGS is identical, some people decide that a precise disease label is of no consequence and that they therefore do not need either a blood test and or an intestinal biopsy.[10]

Many more people want doctors to tell them the cause of their troubles but wait for years to find a physician who will order the requisite tests. According to the University of Chicago Celiac Disease Center, "The average delay in diagnosis for a person with symptoms is 11 years. On average, a child will visit eight pediatricians before being diagnosed with celiac disease."[11] Jerome Groopman's widely acclaimed 2008 book *How Doctors Think* opens with a case in point. A woman he calls Anne Dodge had consulted nearly thirty doctors for her increasingly debilitating gastrointestinal symptoms. She had received diagnoses of anorexia and irritable bowel syndrome but continued to waste away. She also had been treated with four different antidepressants and had undergone weekly talk therapy.[12] Severely malnourished after fifteen years, Anne found Dr. Falchuk, who did something new. He observed her carefully and after reading her medical records took the time to hear her story in her own words. Her narrative convinced him to order a blood test and biopsy, after which he was able to diagnose her with celiac. Like many observers, Groopman faults medical training for physicians' disregard of patients' subjective, or embodied, knowledge. Watching the new crop of students and residents in his hospitals "eye their algorithms and then invoke statistics from recent studies," he concludes that "the next generation of doctors was being conditioned to function like a well-programmed computer that operates within a strict binary framework."[13]

Anne Dodge's story has a familiar ring. During the long interval between the onset of symptoms and a celiac diagnosis, the experiences of patients resemble those of people reporting symptoms of chronic fatigue syndrome, Gulf War syndrome, fibromyalgia, and multiple chemical sensitivities. Like the sufferers of those invisible and "contested" diseases, celiac sufferers report going from doctor to doctor to find relief, receiving a raft of diagnoses and medications, facing widespread skepticism about the existence of their troubles, and watching the quality of their lives diminish.[14] The stories below represent a tiny sample of those recounted in support groups, books, and articles, as well as on blogs and various social media platforms. (Few of these accounts are dated. Because awareness of celiac recently has increased, at least some of the doctors mentioned here might respond differently today. Nevertheless, the narratives provide insight into experiences that, unfortunately, remain common.)

Three years after Groopman's book appeared, Lisa Sanders's column "Think like a Doctor" in the *New York Times Magazine* described a thirty-three-year-old woman who had been disabled by various unexplained pains and mysterious episodes of weakness for the previous ten years. Although she lived in Ohio, her sister sent a letter to a Connecticut doctor, David Podell, who was a friend of a friend, enclosing a letter from the patient that read, "I am very desperate for help. I am struggling every day all day without relief. I have heard you are the best, and if there is help out there, you are the one who will find it. . . . Please give me back my future." In the previous two years she had seen two pain specialists, a gastroenterologist, and an allergist, all of whom had recommended various tests. Reviewing the records, Podell discovered that a blood test had been positive for celiac disease but the gastroenterologist had not considered that diagnosis and did not order a biopsy. After the woman learned to follow a gluten-free diet, her health dramatically improved.[15]

The website of Beyond Celiac, a major celiac organization, reported that the CEO, Alice Bast, consulted twenty-two doctors over eight years before receiving the proper diagnosis. During that period she was weak, suffered from severe diarrhea, joint pain, and migraines that kept her up at night, and had multiple miscarriages. Although five feet nine inches tall, she weighed only 105 pounds and was convinced she had cancer. After a friend suggested that Bast's problems might stem from the food she ate, she agreed to see one more physician. He gave her a blood test. "Sure enough, the results came back positive. After eight years of struggling," she "had her answer: celiac disease."[16]

Social media creators recount similar stories. "My journey to my diagnosis has been a long one," wrote Michelle. "16 years to be precise. It finally ended in May of 2017 with being told I had CD."[17] Alison St. Sure wrote, "The path that led to my diagnosis was long and confusing, typical for many people with celiac disease." In her twenties, "My health started to gradually deteriorate—my asthma worsened, my vision became blurry so I started wearing glasses, and excruciating leg cramps woke me up at night. I was tired at odd times, falling asleep at my desk between classes and in the car on the way home after school. I had tummy troubles but I didn't think it was anything abnormal, even though there were times that I was doubled over in pain." During the next ten years, a host of other painful symptoms emerged. "Doctors didn't know what was causing my severe anemia and gave me a bone marrow exam to test for cancer." The test was negative, "but doctors still did not know the cause of my anemia nor why my list of health problems seemed to be getting longer each year." Finally, when her daily stomach aches were so severe that she had to leave work to lie down in the car, her mother "took things into her own hands. She went on an internet quest to find out what was wrong with me. What she found changed my life. She found celiac disease. I never could have imagined that all my problems could be caused by something I was eating but this was like a bell going off. This was it!"[18] Paula Gardner, cofounder of celiaccorner.com, wrote, "In my case it took several years of symptoms before being accurately diagnosed. My primary care physician suggested I had IBS (irritable bowel syndrome), and alas, never considered—*never connected the dots*—that my symptoms (chronic fatigue, loss of appetite, low iron & folate, 6 months pregnant–looking belly) were all classic celiac symptoms." Even the gastroenterologist to whom she eventually was referred did not initially suspect celiac and instead scheduled various tests to rule out other conditions. Months later, when she began to experience painful lower abdominal spasms, he "*finally*" suggested that she be tested for celiac.[19]

Some celiacs expressed greater anger at the doctors who misdiagnosed them. Ryan, too, had been told he had IBS. "I'm still furious at my doctors for not even entertaining the thought that celiac could be the root cause of all my ills," he wrote on the celiac.com forum. "Given the blood test is so simple it feels almost negligent that they don't run this right at the start to rule it out. . . . Just as well I knew better and kept hitting up Google until my self-diagnosis was proved correct; to think these people get paid highly to be so incompetent makes my blood boil" (November 20, 2020). Gwen had just learned that she had osteopenia (low bone density). "I thought I had worked through the anger that I hadn't been diagnosed years ago (when it wasn't too late to prevent a lot of the issues I have now)," she wrote on the same forum, "but it has raised its ugly head again. My question to all of you is, how did you get past the anger at all the missed/wrong diagnoses over the years? I would have gone back and insisted on the doctor doing something if I hadn't assumed I had IBS for over 20 years. Maybe I could have had children. Maybe I could have prevented the bone loss and hair loss" (October 31, 2017).

Finding the correct diagnosis is crucial for many reasons. First, it confers a medical stamp of legitimacy. "The cognitive and social authority of medicine," remarks sociologist Susan Wendell, "includes the power to confirm or deny the reality of everyone's bodily experience. Thus medicine can undermine our belief in ourselves as knowers, since it can cast authoritative doubt on some of our most powerful, immediate experiences, unless they are confirmed by authorized descriptions."[20] Many sufferers believe that only a definitive diagnosis will convince others and sometimes even themselves that something "really" is wrong. "If I didn't have a diagnosis," one wrote, "I didn't think people would take me seriously. I didn't think that my employer would let me take so many sick days. I didn't think I could be happy until I had a label. While most people fight to reject the labels that are forced upon them by society, I was desperately seeking mine."[21]

A disease label may be especially important for people who have been told they have a psychosomatic illness. Because untreated celiac can lead to depression, some people may indeed have psychological difficulties. But mental illnesses historically have been far more stigmatized than physical ones. Moreover, naming a condition psychosomatic often is tantamount to dismissing it.[22] We saw that Anne Dodge, the woman Jerome Groopman discussed, had been treated with antidepressants and psychotherapy. An ER nurse began, "Like all celiac sufferers, I have a horrendous story to my diagnosis, but the long and short of it being that although psychiatric problems were the first/second/

third thing every GP I've ever been to about the symptoms ever said . . . someone finally listened to me and tested the right thing." She wished she had known about celiac earlier because "I thought I was going crazy with my constant symptoms with no obvious clinical basis, so I just told myself that I was OK and I would just have to live with the constant pain, nausea, diarrhea, vomiting, constipation, teeth problems, nerve problems, etc . . . list goes on." That letter was posted on a blog, where it elicited fifty-three replies, many supporting the nurse's account. One read, "First words out of my GI's mouth after diagnosis? 'You're NOT crazy!' I almost hugged that man! Fourteen years of being dismissed had done a number on my confidence."[23] Actress Jennifer Esposito used some of the same words to describe how she felt when her doctor delivered the news that she had celiac disease: "I had never heard that word before in my life. All the doctors I'd gone to, all the books I'd read in hopes of finding an explanation for my health issues, that word had never popped onto my radar. But I didn't care. She had an answer! All I really heard was: *You're not crazy.*"[24]

A woman who wrote to the celiac.com forum in 2016 had to deal not only with her own doubts about her mental health but also with those of her doctors and family. "In 2010 I went from being the healthiest I have ever been to the next day feeling like I had the flu," Lucinda wrote. "It was as if a light switch was flipped, and it *never* went away. I spent all of 2010 sure I was dying—I was 25 years old and so freaked out. I went to several doctors who all said I was perfectly healthy." One doctor suggested her problem could be fibromyalgia. "I went to another GP to confirm and will never ever forget that day. He told me that I was 'fat' and needed to decide if I wanted to be one of those 'chronic people who spend their lives feeling sorry for themselves' and 'pretending to be sick.' Plus 'fibromyalgia isn't a real disorder and it's all in my head.' I left SOBBING. . . . I have never felt so belittled in my life." In 2014 Lucinda consulted a "gastroenterologist for the unbearable stomach cramps and bathroom issues. . . . He said I had IBS [irritable bowel syndrome] and sent me away. I started to think I was crazy, as did my family. My parents, sisters, husband, all of them thought I was just being dramatic and just had a low pain tolerance. Because there was NO way I could be sick *all the time.*" Finally she visited a psychiatrist. After listening to Lucinda's story, the psychiatrist "felt that something was wrong and was determined to figure it out. She ran a bunch of tests . . . and got me an autoimmune specialist who instantly suspected celiac disease. A month later all tests are back and it is celiac. I feel like writing all of my previous Doc's to prove I *wasn't* crazy!!!" (September 27, 2016).

A celiac diagnosis also provides validation to mothers of young children who have been told (or tell themselves) that problems such as failure to thrive and challenging behaviors result from poor parenting. Casey Wilson, an actress, director, and writer, wrote that when her son lost weight, complained of stomach aches, seemed depressed, and had a seizure, "I beat myself up mercilessly, a stream of cruelty in my head: *If you hadn't been so focused on your career, you would have learned to cook beyond rudimentary fish stick and buttered pasta? You didn't breastfeed enough!*" Although her husband did not blame himself, "I maintained the situation was absolutely dire and it was my fault, that what needed fixing was me." But then, one day, "the results from our son's blood tests were back and we got a call from our doctor. He told us our son had celiac disease." Like many others, she found the name a comfort: "It was a shock, followed by unimaginable relief."[25] Ann Campanella, a former magazine and newspaper editor, noted that when she learned her daughter had celiac, the doctor explained that "despite eating multiple times a day, our daughter was literally starving because her food wasn't nourishing her. *This* is why she was small; *this* is why she was hungry all the time; *this* is why she had trouble sleeping. Part of me already knew this. But to hear confirmation from the doctor was different." For years she had known "deep down there was something despite the myriad times my concerns had been dismissed, rejected, even ridiculed."[26]

Second, a disease label is a prerequisite for treatment. Campanella's daughter's diagnosis initially inspired guilt as well as relief: "A yawning chasm opened within me as I took in the information that Sydney's small intestine had been damaged. Scarred, inflamed, injured. . . . She had suffered, and I hadn't been able to stop it. Could I ever forgive myself?" But now she could take action: "We had proof. We knew what was wrong. We could begin to fix it. My body itched to start the healing process and to go out and find every crumb of wheat that might be in our home and banish it forever." Paula Gardner vividly remembered the doctor's phone call disclosing her diagnosis. She wrote,

> I had just picked the boys up from school and was heading home when I received the call. It was my gastroenterologist informing [me that] I had tested positive for both Celiac and Lactose Intolerance. It was a five minute conversation . . . *but one that changed my life forever.* . . . I questioned if there were any associated complications and he matter-of-factly answered, yes, untreated Celiac could lead to another disease, osteoporosis and cancer. That was all I had to hear—an increased risk of the dreaded "C." *No way* was I going there. Within the next minute, I became gluten-free and I knew it would be for a lifetime—no turning back—there would be no cheating.[27]

Third, the diagnosis enables those who have felt profoundly alone with their problems to discover that they belong to a community of sufferers. Although the blogger who calls himself Gluten Dude later became a fierce critic of the celiac.com website, he recalled how helpful it once had been to him: "It was a resource that people with celiac disease could turn to for guidance and support. They had a forum where people could connect with one another and get answers to questions they had." When he was diagnosed in 2009, he turned to the forum, posted a message, introduced himself, and "felt connected."[28] As we can see throughout this book, the forum has remained a place where celiacs can express their concerns and get help from others. Lucy had lived with celiac for two years by the time she was eighteen. "Finding this message board has really helped me a lot," she commented. "Before I felt so alone" (February 9,

2004). Another entry reveals the kind of emotional support that is available. Maddy wrote that she was "crying and in shock and overwhelmed. I just don't know how to do all this. I feel like I am fighting a silent battle and losing. I don't think I will ever be gluten free." That comment elicited the following replies:

"Oh, you are not alone! We have all been there. Your frustrations and sadness are completely normal. Whose life is going so well that they would welcome a major life problem like Celiac? Nobody's!"; "It is tough and time-consuming to master the gluten free lifestyle; but you WILL be able to do it! One step at a time. Keep reading topics on this site and keep coming back with your questions. This site is loaded with kind and knowledgeable fellow Celiacs who are eager to help you. There is plenty of love and support available here"; "It is normal to grieve! Gluten-free is hard but it gets better! You are not alone!"; "Welcome. It is hard at first. More than a few of us have broken into tears at the grocery store during the first few days or weeks. Some of us also go through a withdrawal which can contribute to the depression and anxiety about all the changes we have to go through. It will get better" (November 4, 2015).

Many people with celiac also join in-person support groups, which have proliferated through the country. Studies find that although in-person groups are most effective, online forums can reduce members' sense of isolation and improve their quality of life.[29]

Concerns

Nevertheless, few people welcome the news that they have celiac. Asked by two interviewers whether he had been relieved to learn he had celiac after eleven years of misdiagnoses, one man answered, "Hell no, I wasn't relieved with the diagnosis, everything I enjoyed eating, I couldn't eat anymore." Other people told the interviewers that they felt "overwhelmed" when they realized that avoiding gluten meant that their entire diet had to change.[30] Comments on the celiac.com forum echoed those sentiments. "This has got to be one of the saddest days for me," Olivia wrote. "Although I think the doctors have finally figured out what's wrong with me, I'm now faced with a life-changing illness that has gotten hold of me at age 28—and I still have my whole life ahead of me. Now, for the rest of my life, all the foods I've enjoyed eating or cooking are making me miserable and I can no longer just be part of the many people who enjoy whatever they want to eat" (February 5, 2015). Emma wrote, "So I was just recently diagnosed with Celiac disease and I am having trouble wrapping my head around it. . . . While I know that maintaining a gluten free diet is going to help me feel better—I can't get over the fact that I cannot eat my favorite foods anymore. No more pizza, no more pasta, no more wheat thins—yes I realize there are gluten free versions of all of these but it's obviously just not the same" (May 26, 2016). Sophia commented, "Changing your eating habits after 30 years is not exactly easy" (November 19, 2016).

Celiacs also worried that their avoidance of certain foods would result in social isolation. "Seems like despite there being some gluten free options in certain restaurants," Paul remarked, "I'm going to be hugely limited in food options. Either sitting on the side looking on or just plain not able to go out much anymore. Already had the first hitting-home moment watching colleagues eating pastries that were brought in while I just have to look on . . . then it dawns that this is never going to get better—urghh." As for dating, he continued, "basically seems game over on that front unlike many who are diagnosed with understanding partners/spouses I'm still in the dating game, which is judgemental enough as it is without all the complications that the gluten issues bring. I've read even kissing someone with lipstick/make-up is apparently a big no-no. . . . Once any dates hear that they won't be coming back. . . . Forever alone status confirmed is how it looks right now" (September 25, 2016). Nora, the wife of a man who had just received a diagnosis, asked ruefully, "How will we ever go to a friend's house for dinner?" (November 21, 2020). Solomon wrote, "I have a girlfriend of another culture and I loved eating her family's food but most of it has gluten. Also, I'm of Italian heritage and now my nonna can't cook all the things she used to for me. I am upset at how this will affect my relationships with those close to me" (July 14, 2020).

Another source of anxiety was the knowledge that a celiac diagnosis increased the risk of other, even more frightening disorders. "I am at the start of what feels like the end of my life as I know it," Timothy wrote. "Been doing nothing but reading for the past week and frankly it's terrifying. . . . Rightly or wrongly right now I see this diagnosis as a death sentence long-term. Looks like it brings other associated illnesses with it. . . . I've only really had noticeable symptoms for the past year or so but wonder how long this has been going on for and what damage has already been done. All seems to have started from when I turned 30 (I knew I was dreading that age for a reason) and right now I wonder how long I'm going to last before the really bad stuff starts" (September 25, 2016). Ann had just learned that her seven-year-old daughter had celiac. "This is all so new," she commented, "and the more I read the more scary it seems" (December 31, 2017). The long wait for a diagnosis heightened Jordan's fears: "After 8 years of being ignored by doc, I finally got my panel and it's official now. I plan to start gluten free diet ASAP[;] however I am scared it's too later [sic] since I have been undiagnosis [sic] for so long. I'm scared right now and cant [sic] imagine leaving my family" (February 28, 2013).

Finally, the forum participants had questions about the dietary prescriptions. Roxanne expressed disbelief at their comprehensiveness: "After a weekend of internet searches and reading everything I can get my hands on, I am in celiac disease overload. I mean COME ON, Chapstick is not OK???????????!!!!!!!!!!! And I need to check my shampoo? Seriously, how important is topical exposure?" (September 15, 2015). A woman who described herself as "new to this gluten free diet" was going to her mother-in-law's house for Thanksgiving: "I am wondering if I can eat the turkey meat if it has been stuffed with gluten bread. My husband and mother in law think it will be fine, [saying] 'just take the breast from the top it won't touch the bread.' But the more I read about cross contamination, the more I am doubting that I can. Any advice would be great" (November 9, 2007).

Many other writers understood the details of the regulations but wondered how rigorously they had to be applied. Jordan asked, "If I have been officially diagnosed and knowingly ingest small amounts of gluten, am I shortening my life? Am I being irresponsible as a patient? Have any of you had these same thoughts? I just really miss my old diet." He concluded, "I was happier before I was diagnosed" (January 24, 2018). Kelly, the mother of a newly diagnosed girl with "relatively minor" symptoms, similarly wondered "how vigilant" they had to be: "Is everyone different and some can tolerate tiny amounts? Or does everyone who has Celiac have to be extremely careful about every little speck of gluten they come across?" (August 4, 2016). Sharla noted that she was "doing all the research" but consulted the forum because she was "just afraid of making a mistake. Is eliminating obvious gluten good enough to start or is it all or nothing?" (November 21, 2020).

Writers who had learned that they had to scour their kitchens and remove every remnant of gluten had still other questions. "So I know that stainless steel pots and pans are okay to use even if they were used for gluten in the past, as long as they are cleaned properly, right?" Jackie asked. "But is there any special way to clean them, or just soap and water and a cloth is fine? What about if your stainless steel pots have scratches though? I was just looking at my pots and I can see little scratches on the bottom inside. I think someone was scrubbing them with something harsh" (April 22, 2015). Marcia wanted to make her kitchen safe for her husband, who had just learned he had celiac: "Suppose bread crumbs fall into the silverware drawer. When you pick out your spoon, there are no crumbs attached. Is that spoon contaminated due to only molecules of gluten that could cling to the surface? . . . Another crumb (and maybe dumb) question. Suppose there are bread crumbs on one end of a stick of butter. The other end is crumb-free. Is that end OK, or not OK?" (November 15, 2015). The mother of a newly diagnosed five-year-old had a question about her knives: "They are stainless steel but have plastic handles. I've read so much about gluten getting into crevices. I'm wondering if I have to replace the knives because of the plastic" (September 7, 2017). Another mother asked, "Can I wash gluten and gluten-free dishes together in the dishwasher?" (November 2, 2016).

Advice

Few medical professionals are equipped to answer these questions. As the University of Chicago Celiac Disease Center writes, "Once diagnosed, people with celiac disease often receive no instruction on the only medical treatment to treat their condition—the gluten free diet. As a result, the newly diagnosed celiac struggles to learn the diet on his/her own, often consuming gluten by mistake and delaying their recovery."[31] Forum participants who had expected their doctors to provide advice were stunned to discover how little was forthcoming. Wendy, for example, wrote, "According to my GI Dr the Celiac Disease is 'pretty severe.' That's it. In the recovery room he says 'pretty severe' and to see him in a month. And to 'go ahead and start the gluten-free diet.' That's it?? The dietician they referred me to is in a Diabetes Clinic" (September 6, 2017). Lauren recounted a similar experience: "I was diagnosed with celiac disease just before Christmas. My GI was NOT very helpful after she told me I had a severe case of the disease, so severe she's never seen levels like mine (like I know what that means.) She literally gave me three pieces of paper that she printed off a website with a few foods to avoid and told me I had to worry about cross contamination. She told me to look somethings up on the Internet then sent me on my way" (January 2, 2006). Rebecca's physicians "didn't say anything besides 'no more gluten'" (November 5, 2015). Brian wished his girlfriend's doctors "were a bit more responsive [because] we're still confused about a slew of things" (September 6, 2017). Camilla wrote on her fiancé's behalf, "Both tests confirmed the worst. It was Celiac. Once diagnosed, that was it. We didn't get a follow up appointment. We weren't referred to anyone to talk about what the next steps were, and how this could affect our lives. We were just thrown out, with this confusing diagnosis, left to fend for ourselves" (July 7, 2014).

One reason for the apparent unwillingness of doctors to dispense nutritional advice is that they know little about the topic. A 2016 study found that interns in medicine, surgery, and obstetrics felt that they had received inadequate training in nutrition.[32] Three years later a *JAMA* article concluded, "Nutrition education in medical school is rudimentary, at best, and limited for the duration of graduate medical education for many specialties. Requirements for meaningful nutrition education in all phases of medical training are long overdue."[33] Another reason is that insurance companies demand an increasingly frenetic work pace. A 2022 study reported that primary care physicians would need to spend 26.7 hours daily to provide the chronic disease management as well as the preventive and acute care that guidelines recommend.[34] As the study's lead author remarked, "If you do surveys with patients about what frustrates them about their medical care, you'll frequently hear, 'My doctor doesn't spend time with me' or 'My doctors doesn't follow up.' I think a lot of times this is interpreted as a lack of empathy, or a lack of willingness to care for a patient. But the reality—for the majority of doctors—is simply a lack of time."[35] The doctors who hurry away after diagnosing celiac disease may know little about the gluten-free diet and operate under severe time constraints.

The failure of physicians to advise celiacs has elevated the importance of dietitians and nutritionists.[36] The American College of Gastroenterology 2022 guidelines about managing celiac disease state that "a visit with a dietitian is mandatory after diagnosis" and that "subsequent visits as needed to reinforce GFD [gluten-free diet] education and adherence should be encouraged."[37] But many physicians do not refer celiac patients to dietitians, and many insurance programs refuse to cover their care. Ivy's rejection enraged her. She recounted her experience on the celiac.com forum:

My doctor's office referred me to a nutritionist, at my request. I called to make an appointment and the nutritionist's office told me to check with my insurance company first . . . and they told me they only cover nutritionists' visits for diabetics! The woman I spoke to had never even heard of celiac disease! Never mind that, like diabetes, celiac disease requires a lifelong medical diet in order to maintain health, and never mind that ABSOLUTELY EVERY resource on the topic says that the first thing any newly diagnosed celiac should do is to run, not walk, to a certified nutritionist. I'm sorry I don't have a more popular disease, but celiacs need health care!! Argh. As you can tell, I'm just about ready to start breaking some skulls (figuratively, of course!)—it's so frustrating to deal with a health care system that exists solely to prevent sick people from getting health care! (June 20, 2005)

In August 2020, US senators Susan Collins and Gary Peters introduced legislation to expand Medicare coverage for dietitian visits for a number of diseases and conditions, including celiac. Subsequently US representatives Eliot Engel and Peter King introduced a companion bill.[38] This legislation could make a difference only if patients are convinced about the value of consulting dietitians and nutritionists. A 2008 study of 154 adults with celiac reported that two-thirds rated their nutritionists positively, compared to half for their gastroenterologists and one-third for their primary care physicians.[39] An exchange on the celiac.com forum, however, indicates that some dietitian care for celiacs has serious deficiencies. In 2015 Hazel asked, "Is going to a nutritionist worth it to make sure I am getting everything I need?" The responses suggested she could find better uses for her time and money. "If you know what you can and can't eat," Ava wrote, "my guess is that you won't get much from a nutritionist." Jack added, "I have never found a nutritionist of much value. We Celiacs tend to know more about our diets than they do." The one person who praised a nutritionist had consulted two. "One was no good. She gave me pages she had printed off the internet," Madison wrote. "The other one was excellent but she was part of the Warren Celiac Foundation in San Diego so she knew celiac. I think it depends on who and where you can find one. You can probably get as much information from the Internet" (January 23, 2015). A 2013 study by the Celiac Disease Center at Columbia University found that consultations with dietitians had no effect on celiacs' quality of life, the severity of their symptoms, or their adherence to the gluten-free diet.[40]

A program launched in 2020 has the potential to improve the guidance dietitians and nutritionists offer people with celiac. In July 2020, the Academy of Nutrition and Dietetics published five modules for a Certificate of Training for Gluten Related Disorders. The titles of the modules are "Medical Aspects of Gluten-Related Disorders and Gluten-Free Dietary Treatment," "Going Gluten-Free: Moving Clients from Diagnosis to Implementation," "Enhancing Quality of Life in Individuals on a Gluten-Free Diet," "Gluten-Free Diet and the Life Cycle," and "Nonresponsive Celiac Disease and Developing Alternative Treatments." Dietitians must complete all five modules to receive the certificate. Two organizations seek to motivate dietitians to take the training. The Society for the Study of Celiac Disease, the professional organization of physicians, nurses, dietitians, and allied health professionals who specialize in the treatment of celiac, offers a discount to new members who have completed the modules.[41] The Celiac Disease Foundation provides grants to dietitians who have done the same.[42]

Conclusion

"Diagnosis is central to the definition and management of the social phenomenon that we call disease," writes the medical historian Charles E. Rosenberg. "It is a ritual that has always legitimated physicians' and the medical system's authority while facilitating particular clinical decisions and providing culturally agreed-upon meanings for individual experience." Rosenberg adds that diagnosis became especially significant in the late twentieth century, as a result of both advances in diagnostic technologies and the "conflation of diagnosis, prognosis, and treatment protocols."⁴³ Those comments help us understand the relationship between diagnosis and physician dominance in celiac care. The development of a serological test and internal biopsy for that disease raised physicians' standing by enabling them to bypass patient accounts and rely instead on markers and pathological changes that cannot be detected by the naked eye. We have seen that many patients assume that doctors alone can confirm their subjective experiences. As a result, they go from one doctor to another until they find one who administers the requisite tests.

But some aspects of the diagnostic process may do little to encourage patients to defer to physicians' authority. Rosenberg ignores the impact of a lengthy period between the presentation of symptoms to a doctor and a diagnosis. The anger that filled the patient accounts above indicates that a long delay in obtaining a diagnostic label can seriously undermine trust. Moreover, doctors were not always the first to consider celiac. In one case, a mother "took things into her own hands," finding the disease classification on the Internet; in another case, the patient went on Google herself; and in two other cases, friends proposed celiac as a possibility.

In addition, celiacs do not rely on doctors for either prognosis or treatment. Because their disease cannot be cured, prognostication is irrelevant. The only therapy is dietary, largely outside physicians' purview. Current guidelines stipulate that physicians should evaluate patients three to six months after diagnosis, one year after that, and then on an annual basis.⁴⁴ The majority of patients, however, fail to receive such care. Many of those who do complain about its inadequacy or irrelevance.⁴⁵

Finally, although Rosenberg stresses the significance of diagnostic technologies, this chapter demonstrates the importance of patients' subjective knowledge. Some people with celiac symptoms refuse to undergo conventional medical testing, relying instead on their own subjective experience. As one patient told two researchers, "I know how I feel."⁴⁶ I have noted that Jerome Groopman stressed that his story about Anne

Dodge demonstrates that physicians' denigration of patients' embodied knowledge can have serious consequences. The doctors who read Dodge's medical records but failed to take the time to listen to her describe her illness could not explain her suffering. Dr. Falchuk was able to order the appropriate diagnostic tests because he first asked her to tell her story in her own words.

Sociologist Steven Epstein cautions us against "valorizing" or "romanticizing" experience as a source of knowledge. He quotes Michelle Murphy, who explains that "it is only through particular methods, rooted historically in time and space, that experience becomes a kind of evidence imbued with certain truth-telling qualities."[47] But honoring embodied knowledge remains essential in medicine, especially as doctors increasingly reduce patients to data gleaned from CAT scans, MRIs, X-rays, and biopsies. That kind of knowledge becomes even more important after diagnosis. Regardless of the extent of medical supervision, the primary responsibility for managing the disease rests with patients alone. Doctors provide little guidance about how to avoid being "glutened," the term the celiac community uses for inadvertently ingesting enough gluten to precipitate symptoms and damage the mucosa. As will see in chapter 7, no diagnostic technology can relieve celiacs of the need to exercise constant surveillance over their bodies, trying to detect any sign of gluten exposure and discover how to respond.

6

Barriers to Adherence

Adherence rates to all medical advice are notoriously low, especially in the case of chronic conditions. According to the World Health Organization, just 50 percent of people with chronic diseases in developed countries follow medical regimens.[1] Studies of adults with celiac disease report widely discrepant rates of adherence, ranging from 42 percent to 91 percent.[2] Because fitting in with peers is so important to adolescents, they are especially unlikely to follow the gluten-free diet.[3]

Some studies warn that "extreme vigilance" to the diet can result in maladaptive eating behaviors and lower quality of life.[4] Because strict, lifelong adherence is currently the only path to recovery, however, a large research literature seeks to find ways to promote it. Most studies focus on individual factors, including knowledge of the gluten-free diet, motivation, a sense of self-efficacy, and membership in a support group or advocacy organization. Although some note the cost of gluten-free food, most ignore the impact of unequal resources.[5]

The health-disparities research that has proliferated since the 1980s demonstrates how systemic injustice translates into what epidemiologist Nancy Krieger calls "embodied harm."[6] A few studies provide insight into structural impediments to adherence. One, published in 2016, reported that celiacs with low incomes are far more likely than those with high incomes to report celiac symptoms.[7] Comments on the celiac.com forum help to explain that finding. Although the participants were overwhelmingly middle-class, a few noted the difficulties of following a gluten-free diet with limited financial resources. "My husband and I are pretty strapped for cash lately," Zoe wrote. "His job is laying off 2,000 people and might close permanently, and unemployment is barely paying our rent alone. I cannot afford $6 loaves of gluten free bread and

$8 for 2 pizza crusts. I really am on a ramen noodle budget right now. Even fruits would be a luxury" (May 31, 2012). Arnold wrote that he lives "below the poverty line so eating special foods isn't an option for me. It's whatever I can afford on food stamps" (August 25, 2021). Harriet's nine-month-old baby, Jimmy, had just been diagnosed with celiac, and she worried that her husband and two older children had the same condition. Jimmy had been "a 'surprise' baby," she wrote, "and we could barely afford the two we already had." The family used food stamps for half their food purchases, but Harriet could not find enough gluten-free items (July 1, 2007).

Two participants relied on food banks. "I am a disabled Veteran and I'm on a fixed income," Gerry wrote. "With how pricey gluten free items tend to get, my food stamps run out fast. So I rely on 2 local food pantries. One of those pantries doesn't seem to care when I tell them I have celiac's disease and can't have any items that contain gluten. It just seems so unfair that over half the items they give me have gluten and therefore don't help me at all" (August 4, 2016). Joan's husband recently had lost his job. "With resources now exhausted," she commented, "we have had to turn to a food bank. You don't get to choose what food you get and they do not make any allowances for dietary needs. 90% of everything they give you is a bakery item. The rest is items that may or may not contain gluten. My husband ate the gluten containing items and saved the gluten free items for me. . . . This however left me with very little to eat" (June 3, 2020).

A few writers noted other ways in which low incomes hindered adherence. "Trying to make my house and home [gluten free] is going to be an impossible task," Lucy wrote. She could not afford to buy all new pots and pans. Moreover, "We don't have the space to make a part of the kitchen gluten free only. Anyone else dealing with the same issues?" She had begun to feel that trying to avoid gluten was "just a waste of time" (May 29, 2012). Jessica lived with her husband in a "rented very tiny home, so small it could be part of the tiny homes movement." She could not keep her food separate from her husband's because the only counter space was the stove top (June 25, 2015). Dennis wrote that he had no control over food preparation because he was homeless and slept on friends' couches (September 13, 2020). Although none of the writers identified themselves as living on the streets, in cars, or in shelters, we can assume that complying with celiac instructions is virtually impossible in those circumstances.

Another study highlighted the impact of living in economically depressed communities. The researchers concluded that one in six people with celiac can be considered food insecure, meaning that they do not have sufficient access to nutritious and healthy food. Fewer than one-quarter of those individuals adhere to the gluten-free diet.[8] Other studies remind us that living in low-income communities that lack supermarkets imposes a special hardship on people with celiac because residents must rely on fast-food restaurants and convenience stores, neither of which is likely to offer gluten-free items.[9]

Celiac advocates have sought to address the issues of poverty and food insecurity in various ways. Some provide advice on eating gluten-free on a budget. (These tend to include such common suggestions as cutting coupons, looking for bargains, eating less meat, shopping in ethnic markets, and cooking in bulk.)[10] The Celiac Disease Foundation has worked with the Los Angeles County Food Equity Roundtable, which seeks to end the food insecurity experienced by various groups, including those with dietary restrictions.[11] In 2023, the CDF wrote a letter signed by twenty-one medical, professional, and nonprofit organizations to the Department of Agriculture urging it to include more gluten-free options in the Special Supplemental Nutritional Program for Women, Infants, and Children.[12] The National Celiac Association has provided a guide for food-assistance organizations explaining why they should offer more gluten-free options for people in food pantries.[13] The Gluten Intolerance Group established a partnership with Cutting Costs for Celiac, a nonprofit organization helping poor families.[14] In addition, various other nonprofit groups either provide gluten-free food assistance locally or ship boxes across the country.[15]

A British study reminds us of the impact of language difficulties on adherence. More than half of South Asians but just 4 percent of Caucasians had difficulty understanding food labels; moreover, celiacs who could not understand labels were less likely than others to adhere to the gluten-free diet.[16] We can assume that a US study similarly would find that reading labels is especially difficult for people who speak little or no English. Although food labels are often hard for English speakers to understand, they are rarely translated and thus virtually incomprehensible for those who are not fluent in the language.[17] Approximately 22 percent of Americans five years or older speak a language other than English at home.[18] Approximately 10 percent of working-age Americans (eleven million people) do not speak English "well."[19]

Institutions

The Gluten Intolerance Group has published a list of suggestions for people planning a hospital admission, including getting a written request for gluten-free food from the physician, calling in advance to speak with people in various departments, informing the nurses of the need for a special diet, reading the menu in advance, and asking to speak to the hospital dietitian.[20] Most hospital admissions, however, originate in the emergency room.[21] As one observer notes, "Hospital cafeterias are not equipped to handle cross-contamination on a whim's notice. A nutritionist or dietitian needs at least a week of advanced notice before you arrive to notify and prepare their chefs and kitchen staff with appropriate directions."[22]

We also cannot know how many hospital personnel honor advance requests—or even understand them. Janice wrote on the celiac.com forum that she wanted to share "a friend's hospital experience because honest to god, it was so bizarre it's hard to believe!" The friend had stayed overnight in the hospital following a C-section. "She'd heard a lot of horror stories about people's gluten free experiences in the hospital, and as she has food allergies on top of the celiac disease, she decided to bring her food and not eat the hospital food." The hospital, however, insisted that she fill out the meal order. Although her form "already had a big 'gluten free' across the top, added by the staff," every meal delivered to her had food containing gluten (March 29, 2012). Other forum participants recounted their own stories. Although Hazel had been told that her surgery to repair an abdominal hernia would keep her in the hospital just for the day, she understood she might have to stay overnight and made plans for her daughter to bring her food. "Well, the best laid plans," she wrote. "Things did not work out as planned and it was a dietary nightmare." She ended up staying overnight but the hospital would not allow her daughter to bring in food. "Long story short," she continued,

> the staff told me I had to eat something before I could leave. The ONLY thing and I do mean the only thing on the menu even close to something I could even risk eating was cream of rice. So I ordered it. The girl brought it and said, "Here is your cream of wheat." Seriously, I mean SERIOUSLY. . . . My Chart said celiac right on it, I told the person that took my order I was celiac and they bring me CREAM OF WHEAT!!!!!! They may just as well served me rat poison!!! I lost it!!!!!!!!!! When the nursing staff was trying to calm me down the RN on duty all but snickered at me when I said I could not eat the eggs on the menu because they had gluten and probably soy in them (powdered eggs because institutions are not allowed to have raw eggs on the premises). (June 23, 2013)

The actress Jennifer Esposito was equally incredulous when hospital staff displayed their ignorance about celiac. Although she wrote "CELIAC DISEASE" in large, red letters on the form she signed before surgery, the recovery-room nurse handed her a tray with saltine crackers, a cup of Jell-O, and a package of juice. When Esposito explained why she could not eat the saltines, the nurse said she had never heard of celiac. "Are you kidding me," Esposito wrote. "I'm in a New York City hospital and they don't know what celiac disease is? I closed my eyes. I wanted to go to sleep for a week. I didn't have the energy to explain. I shouldn't *have* to explain." When the nurse continued to insist that Esposito eat the saltines, she agreed to some water.[23]

Parents of children with celiac in public school are encouraged to seek accommodations for them under Section 504 of the 1973 Rehabilitation Act. Some parents, however, describe disheartening struggles to achieve compliance. Because "everything went well" the previous year, Louise felt confident that her daughter's school would make special plans for the girl again. But the lunchroom staff "said that they couldn't find the food at the store so they couldn't buy them." Louise then found replacements at a local store. "I thought all was going to be fine now," she continued. "The only thing they could not get in town is the bread and pizza. I informed them that I would supply them for her." Nevertheless, the school gave the girl cold cuts for every meal and no bread or pizza. "I have tried every way to make it easy on them," Louise concluded. "But the more I make it easy on them the less they want to do. Can anyone help me in advising me on what to do?" (October 18, 2008). Rachel also met resistance when she tried to file a 504 plan. "I'm trying so hard to not be frustrated," she wrote, "but feel we are getting the run around and not being heard. HELP!!" (August 15, 2019).

Eating safely is even more difficult in institutions requiring long-term residence. Colleges and universities have received the most attention. In 2012, the Department of Justice and Lesley University in Cambridge, Massachusetts, reached a settlement under which the university agreed to provide gluten-free food options in its cafeteria and pay fifty thousand dollars in compensatory damages to students with celiac and food allergies who had been required to purchase meal plans but not provided with enough options they could eat.[24] After a student with celiac disease at Rider University in New Jersey filed a complaint under the Americans with Disabilities Act, the Department of Justice reached an agreement with the university in 2019 requiring it to accommodate students with allergy-related disabilities rather than rely on its food service vendor, make certain that allergen-free food is prepared in special areas, allow students to pre-order meals, and employ a full-time dietitian to advise the university about issues that arise.[25]

Legal action, however, cannot ensure that cafeteria staff receive adequate training, take requisite precautions, and provide gluten-free food that is ample, varied, and nutritious. One Tulane University student told interviewers that "gluten-free dining facilities are A+. . . . Overall, the school provides healthy delicious meals that make being gluten-free in college very easy."[26] Others, however, report different experiences. A Colorado College student stated, "Having worked as a student worker with dining services, I was well aware that there is no allergy awareness for staff. There is no effort to prevent cross contamination for any student, including even simply changing gloves."[27] Gluten Dude posted the following letter from a student who had transferred to a new college as a junior in 2015:

> Before I began this semester, my school assured me that there would be many vegetarian and gluten free options for me. So far there has not. The employees constantly tell me they are out of gluten free products or the preparation of the food is never safe. The gluten free bagels are put in the same toaster as regular bagels, the same cutlery is used, gloves aren't always changed, pans [that] used food that contains gluten are then used for gluten free foods, etc. It's a mess. I have met with my campus nutritionist and the head of our dining halls. They continue to tell me that the issues will be fixed soon, but progress still hasn't been made.[28]

A 2016 survey conducted by the National Celiac Association reported that the difficulty of eating safely at colleges and universities had a "significant, perhaps devastating, social and educational impact" on students "at a point in their personal development when they are particularly vulnerable. First time away from home (and the parental and long term support systems), making new friends, trying to adjust to new social norms, taking on more challenging loads." Then suddenly they "get sick," "have to pre-order food," "have to eat separately from their new friends," "miss classes," "have to advocate for themselves," and "end up paying double for food (no refund on the meal service), no safe cooking facilities, not much more than junk food available outside the cafeteria." More than 70 percent of students with celiac stated that their dietary restrictions had at least a moderate effect on their social lives. One said, "I feel weird and bad when I have to keep being like 'yall I can't eat at any of these restaurants' or not being able to reliably eat at a certain dining hall and people get upset and then I feel like a bad person and sometimes end up going places when I can't eat anything." Another commented, "People do not want to put in that little bit of extra effort to make sure that I can eat and eat safely. They think it's a joke and not a serious medical condition. I've been told to either eat before I go out or bring my own food along because no one else can be bothered to go to a restaurant where I can eat or make sure that I can have a bag of chips at a party." Nearly a third (32 percent) of the respondents stated that the need to locate gluten-free food had at least "some" impact on their educational success. "After being glutened," one student wrote, "the brain fog I experienced often made concentrating in class nearly impossible. Those days I may as well not have been in the classroom."[29]

But if college students can be considered an especially vulnerable group, they have far more resources, alternatives, and clout than nursing home residents and incarcerated people. Finding a nursing home bed is difficult even without a celiac diagnosis. Most facilities have lengthy waiting lists. People who rely on Medicaid, public assistance for low-income Americans, are especially disadvantaged. Because the program's reimbursement rate is very low, most facilities give priority to short-stay patients recovering from acute illnesses, who can rely on Medicare, public insurance for those sixty-five and over, which reimburses facilities at a much higher rate. Nursing homes also seek long-term patients who can pay their own way, at least initially. Medicaid recipients thus must often wait an extremely long time to find a place.[30]

The mother of novelist Curtiss Ann Matlock should have been one of the lucky ones because she was able to rely on Medicare to pay her way.

Matlock's essay, however, demonstrates that the need for gluten-free food exacerbates everyone's access problems. The admissions coordinator of the first nursing home Matlock and her mother toured "proudly proclaimed the facility as being on Newsweek's top recommended list, and gave the appearance of understanding my mother's gluten-free diet. . . . The woman went so far as to take notes of my mother's preferences, her love of sleeping in and drinking coffee, and then plopped in my arms a thick packet of Medicare forms. In all ways she had been exceedingly pleasant." Matlock was thus shocked when the woman called to say that the facility had rejected the mother "because of her diet." The admissions coordinator at Matlock's second choice had no beds available and declined her request to speak with the dietician. The third facility was willing to put her mother's name on the forty-person waiting list but showed little interest in the brochures about celiac Matlock offered to leave. Finally, with the help of a social worker, she found a facility that was willing to accept her mother for a week.[31]

Matlock's mother's first days at her nursing home went well, in part because Matlock hired private caregivers to monitor her food and educate the kitchen staff. "The dietary manager went so far as to voice his gratitude to one of the caregivers for helping them learn what my mother could and not eat." But after Matlock converted her mother to long-term care, "things went downhill." Sandwiches and cake often appeared on her tray. Matlock and the caregivers "consulted with the dietary manager and the kitchen staff. We thanked them for the good food when it came. We explained again what she could and could not have." But one morning Matlock learned that "one of the kitchen staff responsible for following the therapeutic diet said to [the] caregiver: 'Oh, she doesn't need that diet. That's all made up.'" At that point Matlock "faced the fact that my mother was never going to get the food nor the care in eating that she would require at this facility." Matlock decided to bring her mother home and provide care herself.[32]

Talia wrote on the celiac.com forum that because she needed to stay in a rehab facility for a few weeks after surgery, her husband "did quite a search trying to find one that could meet" her dietary needs. "I am at the best available," she continued, "but it's not going well. We met with the chef and he assured me I would be safe. Nevertheless, several mistakes have been made." Although her husband brought her some food, she was losing weight and could not avoid "being glutened" (October 8, 2013). Sarah worried about her mother, who had been sent from a hospital to a rehab facility for a month. A therapist who worked there half-days told Sarah that the staff "are clueless on gluten-free diet." Sarah could bring her mother some dinners but had a very sick husband at home and could not remain at the facility throughout the day. "This is overwhelmingly sad," she commented (February 3, 2022).

Assisted living facilities (ALFs) originated in a grassroots movement in the early 1980s to provide alternatives to nursing homes by granting residents more autonomy and providing less institutional surroundings. As they expanded rapidly in the 1990s, for-profit companies increasingly took control. In 2016, approximately 81 percent of assisted living facilities were for profit; more than 57 percent were affiliated with large chains.[33] Elderly people with celiac commonly report either difficulty gaining admission or a lack of attention to their needs after they enter. Nancy began to worry about her own future when she heard about a friend who was struggling to find a place in an ALF for her mother who had celiac disease in New York. Having read some of the older threads on the forum, Nancy found that residents were told to order the regular option and just avoid the bread (November 27, 2022). Nicole had decided finally to leave her "loveless, emotionally abusive marriage." Because she no longer could live alone, she assumed an ALF would be the best option. "That was before I started talking with a few of them," she wrote, "and realized that they are really not set up to handle a true gluten free diet plus handle other food intolerances. They were all very good intentioned but I hate to put my health in the hands of people who don't really understand the requirements of a gluten free meal as I am very sensitive" (December 14, 2022).

Incarcerated people cannot make such choices. Although the United States has just 5 percent of the world's population, it has 20 percent of the global incarcerated population. Approximately two million people live in the nation's' prisons and jails. A disproportionate number are African Americans and members of other racially marginalized groups.[34] The vast majority of incarcerated people lack access to healthy food of any kind. According to a 2020 report by Impact/Justice, "The current system has unacceptably low standards that sacrifice people's health for the lowest cost and highest efficiency." Most states spend much less than three dollars a day per person for food. Because fresh fruits and vegetables are rare, refined carbohydrates (such as white bread, biscuits, and cake) or fortified powdered beverages are used to stave off hunger. Although many kitchens are unsanitary, they rarely receive inspections.[35] Under such circumstances, people who need special meals fare very poorly.

Because celiac affects 1 percent of the population, we can estimate that the disease affects more than twenty thousand incarcerated people. The Americans with Disabilities Act requires prisons to provide gluten-free food to people with celiac. Although a growing number of prisons have gluten-free options, prisons do not provide those meals to all people who need them. Moreover, few facilities have dedicated gluten-free kitchens or staff trained to cook gluten-free food.[36] In May 2019, a reporter recounted the experience of a man formerly incarcerated in the Oneida County jail in Oriskany, New York. When he requested gluten-free food, he was informed that he needed a doctor's order. Although the doctor's order arrived within a week, the man had to wait another two weeks while the staff learned how to prepare the proper food. The food he finally received was unappealing and occasionally covered in wheat-based gravy. He then was transferred to the Collins Correctional Facility, a medium-security prison in Collins, New York, where he was told that no special trays of any kind were available. Although the facility eventually provided him with gluten-free meals, they consisted largely of rice cakes, rice cereal, and rice.[37] In 2020, Gaven Picciano, a twenty-six-year-old Michigan man with celiac, filed a disability discrimination lawsuit against both the Clark County Jail in Vancouver, Washington, and NaphCare Inc., the for-profit company that provides medical services at the jail, claiming that because the staff failed to provide him with gluten-free food, he lost thirty-five pounds and was so malnourished that he lost consciousness during his three-week jail stay. (The court dismissed the case.)[38]

Conclusion

Even with the best intentions, many celiacs who are poor, live in food deserts, speak little or no English, or reside in institutions simply cannot follow a gluten-free diet. Several groups and individuals have sought to address that issue, supplying gluten-free food to food banks, advocating for legislation to mandate the inclusion of gluten-free products in government assistance programs, and providing advice about finding low-cost gluten-free items and eating safely in hospitals and nursing homes. Because many of the problems are intertwined with class and race, however, these efforts offer only partial solutions. Two pieces of legislation have helped celiacs in educational institutions observe the dietary restrictions—Section 504 of the 1973 Rehabilitation Act and the 1990 Americans with Disabilities Act. But the laws are not self-executing, and some institutions resist compliance.

7

Glutened!

Anyone reading the posts of celiac disease influencers on social media can be forgiven for assuming that adherence to the gluten-free diet is not only easy but highly efficacious. As soon as celiacs stop eating gluten, we are told, troublesome symptoms disappear. Although celiac influencers describe their long, tortuous search for a diagnosis, they insist that once they discover the source of their troubles, their lives dramatically improve. Seeking to earn money by selling various products, they frame celiac as an acute event and tell triumphal narratives.

Studies consistently report, however, that many of those who adopt a gluten-free diet continue to experience symptoms for years.[1] A tiny fraction (approximately 1 percent) of celiacs have refractory disease. Some discover that they have not only celiac but also irritable bowel syndrome and various food intolerances.[2] A few others attribute their difficulties to gluten withdrawal. (Although there is no scientific evidence that people go through withdrawal after eliminating gluten, some celiacs have heard about the condition and believe it affects them.)[3] In many cases, however, the cause of persistent symptoms remains unclear.

Moreover, the clinical response may bear little relationship to the extent of healing of the mucosal lining of the small intestine; influencers who tout the rapidity of their recoveries may still have sustained serious damage to their mucosa. Although most studies indicate that mucosal recovery usually occurs with children diagnosed with celiac, it is less certain in adults. Persistent damage of the mucosa is associated with a higher mortality rate.[4] In addition, celiacs live with the constant threat of being "glutened," the term they use for ingesting enough gluten to trigger symptoms. Even those who rigorously follow the dietary regimen are exposed to significant amounts of gluten; the consequences are often severe.[5] It is thus important to contrast influencers' idealized portrayal of recovery from celiac with other personal accounts.

Social Media Influencers

Social media influencers are people who have developed a reputation for their expertise in certain fields and try to educate others and shape their purchasing decisions. Many began by writing blogs and then moved to various social media sites as they became available; no longer "bloggers," they were now called "influencers."[6] Most are young, attractive women who appear white. They convey a sense of intimacy with their followers not only by posting photographs and occasionally videos of themselves but also by disclosing personal information. Although some claim advanced training in their fields, most derive their authority from firsthand experience. As their numbers have grown, researchers have documented the powerful impact they have on their followers.[7] According to a 2019 report, 50 percent of Internet users follow the recommendations of influencers.[8] A 2017 study found that 16 percent of respondents stated that social influencers had "a high influence" on their food choices.[9] Other studies document the impact of health influencers on patients.[10]

People with celiac disease can choose from an enormous variety of influencers. Collabstr, which defines itself as a marketplace connecting brands and influencers, listed the "top 1,249 gluten free influencers" in February 2023.[11] Here I focus on those who identify themselves as having celiac. Expanding their concern to the entire field of wellness, many provide general advice about lifestyle, fitness, spirituality, and nutrition along with recipes and product reviews.

Like many other influencers, those focusing on celiac disease reflect the impact of the positive psychology movement founded by Martin Seligman. The author of *Authentic Happiness* as well as a host of other academic and self-help books, Seligman established the Positive Psychology Center at the University of Pennsylvania. The center offers courses and training programs and sponsors research on such topics as grit, resilience, positive health, and the science of imagination.[12] The movement has rapidly spread to other colleges and universities. In 2006, 855 students enrolled in Harvard's introductory positive psychology course (sometimes called "Happiness 101"), making it the most popular class at the university that year.[13] Not to be outdone, Yale offered a 2018 course entitled "Psychology and the Good Life," which sought to make not only individual students but also the entire campus happier. With twelve hundred students (nearly a fourth of the undergraduate student body), it was Yale's most popular class ever.[14] Outside academia, articles in mass circulation magazines, TED talks, and such television programs as the *Oprah Winfrey Show* introduce the basic tenets of positive psychology to a large swath of the population. As historian Daniel Horowitz writes, "It is hard to think of an academic specialty at the end of the twentieth century and the beginning of the twenty-first that so fully entered the popular realm and so greatly affected the lives of millions of people worldwide—one that, in effect, became a cultural movement."[15]

Most celiac disease influencers explicitly declare their allegiance to the positive thinking movement. "On my website I take an upbeat approach to living gluten-free just as I do in my life," writes Erin Smith, the creator of Gluten-Free Globetrotter.[16] Alison St. Sure of surefoodsliving.com asserts, "My philosophy is to take a positive outlook on the gluten-free or allergen-free diet, while addressing the difficult challenges they present."[17] The subtitle of "Gluten-Free Optimist" is "a positive slice of gluten-free life."[18] Most point to their own experiences to explain why optimism is warranted.

Seeking to develop a sense of intimacy with their followers, celiac influencers claim to understand the challenges of living with the disorder. They often begin by describing their long, difficult search for a diagnosis but then maintain that once they adopted a gluten-free diet, everything suddenly and dramatically improved. "Pam" waited fifteen years for a diagnosis, but then "within two weeks of going Gluten-Free I felt like a NEW PERSON! I had more energy, zero tummy problems, and just felt better overall." The diet also cured her infertility problems: "Two months after going Gluten Free, we got pregnant with twins!"[19] "Lindsi," of bestglutenfreebeers.com, was twenty-two and a year out of college when she learned she had to eliminate gluten. She had one final meal, eating everything she no longer could eat again, "a homemade white lasagna with 2 different types of home-smoked cheese, and BEER. It was a heavenly meal." But the next day she "cut them both out and never went back." Within a month she was "a completely different person. My moods stabilized, my migraines vanished, and my neck pain began to slowly fade. This led to my being able to sleep again at night. My immune system began to improve immediately too." Now she gets "sick like a normal person and only once or twice a year."[20] Although Alison St. Sure described her ten-year ordeal obtaining a celiac diagnosis, her story did not end there. After changing her diet, she "experienced dramatic physical and mental changes. Some occurred immediately, some within a few months, and some a year, but ALL of my health problems that had been plaguing me for so long *disappeared*." Those included two that were unrelated to celiac. Not only did she have more energy than ever before and no more stomach pains, but she also "stopped taking all asthma medication (really!) and stopped wearing glasses (really!)." She concluded, "It was like new life had been breathed into my body as every health problem I had went away. It was truly life-changing."[21]

Moreover, the writers' lives remained full despite the new dietary requirements. A few years after learning she had celiac disease, Kelly Courson "made a crazy fun new friend at work in New York City, Kim Danyluk, and it turned out she was also gluten-free!" The two women "had so much fun making treats for each other, sharing scoop[s] about new products, and discovering new hip gluten-free friendly places to dine." But when they consulted the available books and online resources, they were disappointed. "We sort of wished there was more enthusiasm. We felt there was room on the internet for a site that was informative and entertaining that would help people deal with adapting to and living a gluten-free diet. We personally knew that it didn't have to be a drag!" And so, in August 2003, they launched the blog *Celiac Chicks*.[22] The suggestions Erin Smith posted on "gluten free globe trotter" were "about not only living, but thriving with Celiac Disease."[23] Another world traveler, "Jen," commented, "I am living proof that celiac disease is not the end of my adventures, travels, or fun. I've been to 25 countries with celiac disease! Celiac has only given me more resilience and determination to explore and live an amazing life despite dietary restrictions. My celiac diagnosis story makes me stronger, not weaker."[24] Paula Gardner also expressed gratitude to the diagnosis for engendering personal growth: "Living a gluten-free lifestyle has opened up an entirely new way of eating (& cooking) for me. While meticulously reading labels looking for the absence of gluten, I also discovered how many unhealthy ingredients are *added*—preservatives, dyes, etc. I am now buying less processed, fresher & primarily organic food for the entire family. I experiment with gluten-free baking flours . . . that I never knew existed!" Despite the new challenges she faced, she concluded, "Ultimately, my diagnosis of Celiac has proven to be a serendipitous blessing!"[25]

Now these influencers want to empower others. "Isn't it time to have a gluten-free life that works?" asks Jennifer of Glutenfreemarcksthespot.com. "You're probably *tired* of being afraid to leave the house (too far from the bathroom with all the bloating and gas!), passing on fun celebrations with family and friends, and, especially, missing out on your son scoring the winning goal in the soccer tournament! **It's time to change all that!**"[26] Erin Smith has traveled throughout the world while remaining gluten free. With her new website, Gluten-Free Globetrotter, she seeks to provide "motivation for those with Celiac Disease to get up and live their lives and not be scared of anything. Yes, being gluten-free can be a very daunting life experience, but I encourage you to embrace your gluten-freeness and not limit yourself. If only one person is inspired by this website to step outside of their comfort zone and to do something as simple as try a new restaurant or something as radical as backpacking through Asia, then I will have completed my task."[27]

The exuberance and good cheer pervading these websites help them serve as a giant marketplace.[28] Many endorsements focus on taste and texture. For example, Jenny Levine Finke of Good for You Gluten Free writes, "If you're looking for store-bought gluten-free ravioli options, I've got you covered with a few brands making this once-impossible dish possible again." One brand she tried was Cappello's Gluten-Free Ravioli, "and let me tell you, the taste and texture are incredible. The ravioli held together well and offered up a chewy texture." Although Jenny's kids loved the five-cheese ravioli, she found "the gluten-free butternut squash ravioli . . . unbelievably delicious; I had to stop myself from eating the entire box. The noodles hold together well, and the butternut squash ravioli is seasoned to perfection."[29]

Linking the gluten-free diet with other forms of wellness, many influencers earn money not only by promoting gluten-free food products but also by selling a vast array of goods calculated to improve celiacs' lives, including cookbooks, travel guides, food items, kitchen utensils, and aprons and other clothes, as well as cooking classes and coaching services. Julie Rosenthal wants to help people become more grounded and spiritual, not just gluten free. She introduces gooddiegoodieglutenfree as a "wellness website devoted to clean eating, healthy gluten-free & dairy-free recipes, and holistic wellness."[30] For $190 she provides a sixty-minute coaching session offering "spiritual health tips or quick soulful inspiration" as well as "help transitioning to a gluten-free lifestyle." The month-long package "Rebuild and Glow" costs "$695 and includes a 90-minute session, a 60-minute follow-up session, notes following each appointment, email and text access, and weekly self-care exercises, guided meditations, and bedtime rituals."[31] Karina Allrich, the creator of Gluten-Free Goddess, not only posts gluten-free recipes but also offers a whole line of clothing (including various T-shirts, sweatshirts, aprons, and even a thong), as well as assorted necklaces, mugs, drinking glasses, bags, pillows, blankets, magnets, and journals. All can be inscribed with the name "Gluten-Free Goddess" or alternatively with such phrases as "Gluten Is the Enemy," "Gluten Sucks,"

"Somebody I Love Has Celiac," and "Gluten Puts Another Nail in My Coffin," in a variety of scripts.[32]

The Long Road to Recovery

Although Gluten Dude acknowledges that he qualifies as an influencer, he posts what he calls "rants" in place of enthusiastic testimonials. The following letter appeared on his blog in 2012:

> When I got my celiac diagnosis, after a year of not feeling well, I ASSUMED I would start feeling better if I just stopped eating gluten. Much of what I read online led me to that conclusion. But like many things with celiac disease, assumptions and reality are two very different things. I have been living with my Celiac for three years now, and I continue to be amazed and frustrated with this disease. The havoc it can wreak, and the curve balls it can throw, constantly keep me on my toes. As soon as I think I have the diet down, something slips by me and I get sick. As soon as I think I know exactly what being "glutened" looks like in my life, I get a new or changed symptom.

The letter writer had been led to believe it would "take a year [to] get everything under control and get my life back to the way it was before my Celiac triggered." Now she understood: "My life will NEVER be the same."[33]

Comments on the celiac.com forum echoed those complaints. "I've got a little issue," Anthony began:

> I was diagnosed with celiac last year around June and I used to get the worst stomach aches ever, no one could possibly imagine. I went on a gluten free diet and started feeling better bit by bit. The doctor said I should feel completely better by around September and have no issues with stomach aches, etc. It's been a year since this so-called September, actually a year and two months. I can't find the problem. I never eat out

> because I'm really paranoid about eating gluten but to this very day I found going to the toilet to be a very irregular gamble. It's really difficult to go out and enjoy myself because I do get these random stomach aches that hurt so much. My stomach aches seem to get better then worse then slightly better then worse again. (November 27, 2012)

Ava had received a celiac diagnosis at the age of forty-four, thirteen months before she wrote. Although her stomach problems were now less severe, she had little energy. "I simply fail to understand," she wrote. "Prior to diagnosis I was not as lethargic and fatigued as I am now without exerting myself. I was a working lady at the time.... I used to manage all my chores but now everyday is a nightmare for me. Sometimes I want to go back on gluten as I am fed up with this miserable feeling" (April 23, 2016). Madeline's husband also had been diagnosed the previous year. "At first we thought 'hey, this won't be too bad—we just need to buy more fresh whole foods and things labeled as gluten free—piece of cake!' WRONG!" Although they had eliminated dairy as well as gluten and were very careful about cross-contamination, the husband was "still suffering from celiac symptoms" and had "even progressed to NEW symptoms he never had before his diagnosis and new gluten-free diet." She concluded, "Going through all of this and living such a restrictive life style is so deflating for him when he isn't seeing any improvement and is actually feeling worse" (January 19, 2015).

More than anything else, the constant fear of being glutened challenges the complacency of social media influencers. As already noted, a very high proportion of celiacs who adhere to the gluten-free diet are exposed to gluten and experience symptoms. Questions about glutening filled the celiac.com forum, reminding us both how central that experience is in celiacs' lives and how little guidance they receive about coping with it. Over and over participants asked, Does everyone respond in the same way to having been glutened? (Among the various symptoms writers reported were fever, bloating, headaches, digestive problems, muscle tension, joint pain, abdominal pain, canker sores, anxiety, and depression.) Do individuals experience the same symptoms each time they are glutened? How can you tell if you've been glutened if you are asymptomatic? How soon after exposure do symptoms emerge? A mother wondered if her daughter's stomach problems could have been caused by something she ate thirty-six hours earlier. "Is it possible that the reaction can be delayed this long?" she asked (June 6, 2018). A man recalled that he had begun to feel ill even before he left the restaurant. How soon can one expect to feel better? Penelope wrote that she "got glutened by something this past weekend. Three or four days later I am STILL struggling with severe GI pain. I am getting sharp pains, bloating, and cramps no matter what I eat. I am trying to eat healthy, bland, safe foods. Do other people experience this? Is it normal to continue to experience GI pain for this long? I just want to be sure I'm not re-glutening myself or getting sick from something new, rather than it's still the original glutening hurting me and I need to work it out" (July 9, 2014). Others had questions about possible remedies. Should they try broth, digestive enzymes, probiotics, green tea, supplements, fasting? Is it OK to exercise? And how can you be sure that symptoms stemmed from gluten ingestion rather than another condition, such as food poisoning, stomach flu, or a new food intolerance? In the absence of professional advice, the forum moderators drew on their own experiences to try to answer these questions.

Some forum participants acknowledged that they intentionally consumed gluten. A few could not resist temptation. Since her diagnosis two months earlier, Melinda had not "been able to remain gluten free for more than two weeks. I always make excuses and tell myself that I will start 'tomorrow.'" During the previous year, when she had assumed she was gluten intolerant, she had had no trouble avoiding gluten because she had assumed "it was only a temporary thing." She felt differently after learning she had celiac. "As many of you all know it is mentally very difficult to accept that you have to restrict yourself from foods you love forever. I am Mexican and food is a central part of our life and family traditions, making it even more difficult. To make matters worse, my family owns a bakery that is next to my house so the kitchen is constantly filled with gluten treats, cakes, cookies, everything" (January 14, 2018). Evelyn was now sixteen and had been diagnosed with celiac disease three years earlier. "I don't follow my correct gluten-free diet as I am supposed to and Ive [sic] tried many times to quit," she confessed. "I think I've tried 5 times or more and it works for about a week or less. I don't know what I can do to help me stop cause no one else around me has the same thing. I dont [sic] know anyone at all who shares the same struggle" (January 8, 2015).

A few others had wanted to test their reactions. "I have been dealing with being gluten free," Louis wrote, "a frustrating process as you all know. I just want to eat and not worry what is in it. The other day I did just that, [convincing] myself I could eat [a certain item]. Well I paid over and over" (April 12, 2007). Sadie "had been extremely careful about anything I eat, drink, and even prepared for my husband. We have completely stopped eating out. I went through my kitchen and gave away or threw out all of my plastic containers." Nevertheless, she had had "a self inflicted relapse earlier this year (I just had to see if I had been misdiagnosed, how far I could push things)" (October 22, 2016). Arnold could not exercise his customary vigilance in a crisis. Diagnosed a year and a half earlier, he had "been trying to make this gluten free diet work as well as possible. [But] my son broke his arm and during the trip to the ER, we stopped and I was glutened by what I think was cross contamination from fries because it was late and the place was getting ready to close" (February 20, 2016). Two women had tried to avoid offending their hosts. Carole began to experience symptoms after she ate "4 bites of lasagna at a party the other night when I needed to be polite" (August 20, 2009). June had thought she was safe eating at the house of a friend who had asked June what she could eat. But when June arrived and inquired about the marinade on the flank steak, she learned it contained soy sauce. "I didn't want to be rude," she wrote, "so I ate the steak. (I am not sure what got into me, I NEVER knowingly ingest gluten!! But I did)" (October 1, 2008). As we will see, other celiacs eat food containing gluten in an attempt to conceal their diagnosis.

Like other people with celiac, the participants were glutened inadvertently far more often than they ate gluten deliberately.[34] Because the interval between gluten ingestion and the onset of symptoms can vary, many celiacs have difficulty determining exactly when exposure occurred. "Somehow the dark power of gluten has once again returned to the land," one forum participant announced. "But I don't know. Despite being careful, despite rarely if ever eating out, having given up drink, cooking from one pan etc., etc., I still don't know what it was that I've eaten that's caused this. And that's what's driving me up the wall" (June 23, 2016). Donna "had been feeling pretty well once going gluten free. Joint pain disappeared. Stomach pain disappeared. Indigestion was a lot better, although I still had a little." But "now I'm back to square one. I have spent the last 2 days with stomach pain. Last night, I was doubled over. All day—stabbing pain. I keep thinking, what did I eat? . . . It's just so frustrating" (November 10, 2015). Tim complained, "Seems even buying only foods labeled gluten free and supposedly gluten free is not always enough, and even the most cautious of us can have stuff happen. I have yet to narrow down the exact source but it was something in my pudding/ice cream/shake base that I use for keeping weight on" (February 14, 2017). Eliot wrote, "For the past month I've been having gluten headaches, eczema and canker sores and cannot figure out where the hidden gluten is. I switched dish washer detergent but that is really the only thing I've changed. I've scoured my medications and bath/body products, looked at every food label, kept a food journal, don't eat out, and still can't come up with the culprit. Does anyone have any detective trips to share?" Charlotte noted that she was "racking my brains" to discover the cause of her symptoms (June 20, 2020).

Participants who could identify the cause of their exposure pointed to two major sources. One was the difficulty of reading food labels. A 2020 study found that celiacs frequently encounter challenges identifying gluten-free food. Some result from "misleading labels," others from "erroneous label reading."[35] Although some forum participants had trouble distinguishing between the two, most placed the responsibility on one or the other. Carla believed the fault lay with improper labeling: "My whole body aches, muscles twitch, my lower left abdomen was hurting yesterday and no energy. It makes no sense since I am extremely careful. I bought a gluten free salad dressing but I think it was not gluten free although they labeled it as such" (October 10, 2016). Phyllis had felt safe purchasing a box of tortillas because the label claimed they were both gluten free and wheat free. But when she became ill, she "did a search only to find these brown rice tortillas were recalled in Canada for having wheat in them and the 'filtered water' they use in their other products contains barley! I'm so mad right now" (February 13, 2011).

Celiacs who are unsure about the safety of a particular product are encouraged to contact the manufacturer. Scarlett sent an email to a company after adding onion power to her dinner. "They told me it's not gluten free, they add starch to it," she wrote. "And on the package it was saying we don't add anything else." Moreover, she had found the powder where "they were selling a range of gluten free products. Ugh, Im [sic] so tired of getting glutened by random and useless stuff like this[.] I was doing great for more than a month, then this happened. Im [sic] just extremely sad" (October 23, 2017). Hannah's experience contacting a manufacturer was less productive:

> I've called a few different companies to verify if their product is gluten free. I get the feeling that they just say yes without knowing where gluten can hide. For instance, I called the number on the Wishbone salad dressing as it contains caramel color. As I understand it the caramel color can be a hit or miss with the gluten factor. The woman I spoke with seemed nice enough but didn't sound familiar with my question. She did tell me that all their products are gluten free. Is there any guarantee that these people are providing accurate information? (September 15, 2009)

The moderator responded, "When you call a company, you are speaking with a customer service representative, not a dietitian. In most cases, all they can do is read you the information that they have been given" (September 15, 2009). Another participant complained that food companies "often give us dodgy and vague nonanswers written by lawyers" (June 22, 2015).

Two writers blamed their symptoms on Frito-Lays chips. "I'm kind of new to this," Oliver wrote, "and wondered about reading the labels on food. Can processed food contain gluten even if the label doesn't list wheat or any of the other ingredients that can contain gluten? I had a bad reaction to Frito-Lay's sour cream and onion potato chips, but nothing was listed on the label and on their website it says they're gluten free, although it doesn't say gluten free on the package" (June 13, 2010). Sheila was enraged. "A few hours ago for lunch," she wrote, "I made myself a plain burger. I ate that with Heinz ketchup. I know this is safe as I have eaten it a million times. I usually eat Lays plain Stax but since reading Lays gluten free list, I decided to try Lays Classic plain chips. Within an hour of eating the chips, I got my normal reaction, short of breath, flushed face, extreme bloating and D [diarrhea]. I suspect that Frito Lays has a huge CC [cross-contamination] issue going on. It just makes me furious that some companies claim products to be gluten free and then we get really sick" (March 1, 2011). The confusion Oliver and Sheila experienced might have been expected. In 2015, four and five years after their complaints, PepsiCo's Frito-Lay North American business announced that after consulting with the Food Allergy Research Program of the University of Nebraska–Lincoln, and the Celiac Disease Foundation, it had developed a validation process for testing products labeled gluten free to ensure that they contained less than twenty parts per million of gluten. In addition, the company had added a new, clearer label on the front of certified products as well as a statement on the back.[36]

Many other participants faulted themselves for their lack of caution. "Well, I did it again," Avery wrote. She had been too tired in the morning to read ingredients properly. "I could kick myself," she added (November 20, 2012). Grace had ordered a gluten-free pizza from Domino's, although she "knew it was a risk." (Since 2012, boxes of Domino's gluten-free pizza have displayed prominent warnings that the items are not safe for celiacs.)[37] "BIG mistake," Grace continued. "I had the pizza on Monday afternoon and at 2:30 am Tuesday morning I was woken by a severe headache, which morphed into a migraine, and then some of the symptoms, stomach pain, bloating, nausea. It's now Thursday and I still feel awful, will it get better soon?" (June 23, 2021). Bess had finally started to feel better on her new diet. "Then on Halloween night," she wrote, "I accidentally ate a twix bar (not thinking of the wafer inside the bar) and I swallowed it and thought, 'crap—this has wheat in it!' I had that one bite and threw it away. The next morning I woke up and my eyes were swollen and my stomach was in knots all day! I have never felt pain like that in my life before" (November 4, 2007). Judy, too, had reveled in her new sense of well-being after eliminating gluten from her diet. But the previous weekend she "was eating some Walkers Crisps in a bar, which I knew are 'made in a factory that includes gluten,' but I thought the risk would be minimal—I'm trying so hard to be 100% gluten free, constantly refusing to eat out with people, eat at their houses, etc. and yet somehow every month I make a mistake and lose pretty much a whole week to feeling awful and unable to work" (June 3, 2016). Even the most rigorous adherence to the celiac dietary restrictions could not shield Judy from occasional gluten exposure.

Some participants realized too late that they had to check the label every time they purchased a product. The week before writing, Zack "had been super excited" because he had found Merci chocolate in the store. Then he "did the stupidest thing." He remembered to read the label only after eating several bars (November 5, 2016). Deirdre wrote, "Well it is currently 4:15 am and I am wide awake in a state of full-fledged glutening. It wasn't someone or something else that got me this time but it was me. Ugh. I have no one to blame except myself!!" She had bought a bag of crisps, assuming "that this flavor was gluten free because several others say it right on the bag. I had failed to actually read the label. I had gotten lazy!!!" (October 13, 2008). Elana wrote,

> So almost a YEAR ago, I started purchasing a trail mix that had a good price and I liked. I checked ingredients back then and it had nothing gluten and no warning. I noticed the label changed a while back, but didn't think twice about double checking ingredients. Today I get the idea to look at it, and yup, says it might have trace amounts of things including wheat/gluten. Well I'm such an idiot. Should always check labels. I ate the dang stuff nearly every day. Kids are finishing up my last package as we speak. I can't believe I did that. You'd think with 9 years' experience I'd know better. I feel like a fool and I'm so mad at myself. (July 22, 2017)

Because restaurants were excluded from the Food Allergen Labeling and Consumer Protection Act, they represent the second major source of glutening. A vast array of guides both in print and online help celiacs find establishments serving gluten-free food. In addition, both individuals and groups provide tips for eating out, including choosing restaurants carefully, calling ahead, informing the wait staff of dietary restrictions, selecting simple dishes, without sauces, or salads, and confirming orders after they arrive. But there are few safeguards. A 2018 meta-analysis of studies of restaurant and food-service workers in the United States and Britain identified "many knowledge gaps" about food allergies and celiac disease, "suggesting a need for increased education and training."[38] The following year Columbia University researchers published the results of a study using a portable gluten detection device to test the content of restaurant food labeled gluten free. Nearly a third (32 percent) of the food tested positive; that figure included 27 percent at breakfast and 34 percent at dinner. Gluten was found in more than half of the pizza and pasta tested.[39]

In 2012 Gluten Dude posted a letter from a woman who had ordered from the gluten-free selections at a highly recommended restaurant in Charlotte, North Carolina. Because the waiter could not answer the woman's questions about gluten and cross-contamination, she asked to speak to the manager. "The manager answered the questions right, indicated that they were trained in safety, and told me [the] hamburger was cooked on a separate area. She also added that their GF hamburger buns were the tastiest she had ever had." Before taking a bite, however, the letter writer noticed that her bun "looked just like everyone else's." She thus called the manager back "to question and sure enough, I had the regular bun. I then had to go into a LENGTHY description of why they could not take that burger and merely switch buns. She seemed annoyed. Ultimately my trust was blown so I watched my husband, our daughters/spouses, and my granddaughter eat while I held the four-month-old granddaughter and ate nothing."[40]

Others recounted similar incidents on the celiac.com forum. Amelia's health had improved after eliminating gluten three years before she wrote. "Then one day I went to my tried and true-trusted restaurant who are normally extremely good about preparing gluten-free foods. I ordered the burger on a gluten-free bun. Hooray! I was starving, so when it came, I chowed it down. About 3 bites in I thought, 'Dang, this is awesome, this bun tastes so good.' Then it hit me, oh no. This isn't a gluten-free bun is it. So I asked and it definitely wasn't. . . . A couple days later I started having all the normal symptoms, rashes, abnormal bowel movements, foggy head, fatigue, depression, etc." (August 31, 2013). Carla described herself on the forum as "a newly diagnosed celiac, just about two months into recovering." She "was feeling soooo much better and my bowels were almost back to normal. Well—then my husband and I went out to eat this weekend to celebrate our 10 year anniversary. They seemed very knowledgeable and concerned with cross contamination. About 15 hours later I got incredibly sick" (September 22, 2016). Celiacs often are advised that more expensive restaurants will take greater precautions than less costly ones. Cora discovered, however, that she could not trust the "very nice expensive restaurant" where she ate with her husband and a few friends: "I discussed my meal and the menu with the chef and showed him my celiac card with all the explanations of what is allowed and not allowed. I had a delicious meal of swordfish, Yukon potatoes, tuna sushi w. wasabi, and crème brulee for dessert. We got home around 11 pm and by 2 am I was vomiting and had diarrhea and was shaking, sweating, tachycardiac. . . . This was not food poisoning. Others ate what I ate and no one was sick but me" (August 7, 2006).

Many other participants placed the burden of responsibility on themselves. "Against my better judgment," Carla wrote, "I went out on a limb and headed to Chick Fil A for lunch. They were so knowledgeable and friendly. They confirmed that they used separate fryers for fries of a guest that identify with gluten issues. They even knew exactly what I could and couldn't have on the menu. I was ecstatic! I got back to work, enjoyed my tasty lunch, and 30 minutes later it hit me like a ton of bricks. I was nauseous, my tummy was so loud and I was in pain! Since then I've been foggy headed and emotional" (January 26, 2016). Arthur wished he had trusted his instinct that the restaurant chosen for a birthday party could not be trusted. He had ordered from the gluten-free menu but did not "have the best feeling if it was really gluten free" (January 30, 2017).

Others faulted themselves after servers made mistakes. "AAGGHHH!!!" Savannah began.

> I rarely eat out but I was out with some friends—expected to leave to eat at home, but it went long, so I got brave and ordered cheese and gluten-free bread. The restaurant has a good reputation for being careful with their gluten-free foods and other dietary issues. I should have just eaten the cheese since I know that's always safe, but I was too hungry and lost my good judgment and willpower. Also I haven't had any bread since my diagnosis, so didn't really realize for a bite or two that the bread I had was regular bread. Once I clued in that the bread was too soft, I asked the waitress (had been really clear about the gluten-free bread when I ordered) and she was barely apologetic. OMG. I left immediately to get home before the symptoms started. (January 23, 2015)

Connie similarly held herself responsible for her troubles. "Well I've done it," she wrote.

I've been glutened. Although I've been exceedingly careful with restaurants, I went to a Korean place I trust—the owner herself spoke to me at length about the measures they take to ensure their gluten-free items are gluten free—and chose poorly. In the past I'd always ordered items that had little chance of being mixed up with gluten ones, ones that had just whole ingredients. This place doesn't use wheat-based soy sauces, so they're pretty safe. This time, I made a mistake and ordered these rice sticks. Turns out the server, although I emphasized that I had celiac, and she acknowledged it, failed to make sure that I got the gluten-free version. I didn't even know they had a version that had wheat. (February 1, 2015)

Eden wrote, "Stupid me." Recovery had been going well, but then she "got careless." She and a friend "got together for dinner, it was the third anniversary of the passing of our closest friend. We went to the only restaurant close to me that I would eat at. I got the same salad I had in the past and garlic fries which I have had also. Since I never go out I had forgot that they serve bread with the salad, and they brought it out with two slices of French bread sitting on top of my salad. I should have politely sent it back and asked for a new salad. Did I do that? NO! My friend ate my bread and my salad which had been contaminated!" (August 31, 2013). Eden's symptoms began shortly after she left the restaurant and worsened the following day.

Conclusion

The relentlessly cheerful tone of celiac influencers undoubtedly provides reassurance and promotes the sale of various products, but it offers little insight into the challenges of trying to recover from celiac. Influencers pay scant attention to the many people whose symptoms fail to abate as soon as expected, or ever. Evidence about the prevalence of gluten exposure and the harm it can cause reminds us that, far more than the positive attitude or sense of adventure influencers encourage, celiacs need a high level of vigilance to stay safe and even then cannot always do so.

8

"An Alien in a Strange World"

Living and Working with Celiac Disease

Although a critical concern of medical professionals is to increase celiacs' adherence to the gluten-free diet, the principal fear of newly diagnosed patients is that the disorder will undermine their work lives and fracture their social relationships. That fear often is realized. A rich body of literature demonstrates that social connectedness is essential for maintaining mental and physical health.[1] Because social, religious, and family events often revolve around food, however, many celiacs find themselves isolated and alone when they are most in need of practical and emotional support. Most people with celiac can remain in the labor force, but many take time off to cope with symptoms. Without accommodations at work, they experience serious economic repercussions. Although several studies explore the effect of celiac on social activities, the impact of the disease on labor force participation remains largely unexamined.[2]

Social Disconnectedness

A study published in 2008 found that, to maintain the gluten-free diet, 44 percent of the 154 respondents with celiac avoided eating away from home and 21.4 percent avoided social engagements.[3] It is thus unsurprising that a central theme of comments on the celiac.com forum is the pain of loneliness and its detrimental effect on mental health. Rosemary wrote that she was trying various ways to deal with her depression, but "the celiac isolation is making it so hard to combat the blues. I just learned I wasn't invited to [a] family function because they didn't want to worry about my diet (even though I bring my own). This seems to be the trend. My friends don't have me over anymore and now my family is excluding me. This disease is so hard mentally" (June 14, 2013).

More commonly, celiacs intentionally withdraw from social engagements. Donna explained why she had no use for the positive psychology movement. "I know we're supposed to be positive," she wrote, "and the big message whenever anyone gets a diagnosis of any sort is 'Don't let it stop you from living your life!' or some such positive line to live by! Well," she continued, "I've found that in the 8 months since my whole family has been diagnosed, I'm a heck of a lot happier if I lay low, avoid attending food related functions, skip the road trips to stay with family, etc. Is that bad?" (September 15, 2014). Those who already had removed themselves from social events stressed the loneliness that ensued. Lisa, for example, was "concerned" because she seemed to "have had to become increasingly socially and professionally isolated, and this seems to be contributing to some depression. I no longer attend work events where food is served, go to bars or restaurants, or attend professional conferences" (May 16, 2016). Marilyn commented, "I can withdraw even more into my own safe gluten-free bubble but I'm already feeling cut off from being able to socialize like I used to and that's making me depressed and isolated" (June 3, 2016). Georgia, the mother of young children who had just received diagnoses, wrote, "I'm terrified of going anywhere or doing anything. I worry that my kids are going to accidently get gluten somehow and I have become a recluse!" (April 7, 2015).

Other forum participants complained of feeling alone and unsupported because they lived with people who failed to respect the celiac dietary prohibitions. Audrey was the only member of her household restricted to a gluten-free diet. "Everything appeared to be going alright," she wrote, "until recently when I did some observation during my time off." She watched her husband "getting out his bread to make a sandwich, then he opened up the lunchmeat/cheese and grabbed what he wanted, made his sandwich, sealed it up and put it away. . . . When I asked him not to do that or at least wash his hands after the bread and before opening/closing the packages, his response was, 'I'm only touching what I am going to eat.' Don't get me wrong, he is understanding, takes this seriously, I just didn't realize he was taking shortcuts" (June 26, 2009). Cecilia's complaints also focused on her husband: "He leaves his crumbs all over the kitchen and will regularly cut his gluteny bread on my cutting board. Which has deep ridges in it and there is NO WAY I can get all the gluten out. I told him I'm buying myself a new cutting board, and he says that I am being ridiculous and wasteful, since washing it should be enough, and we can't afford to keep buying new stuff because of my paranoia" (September 14, 2006).

There are various ways to understand the challenges these celiacs encountered interacting with family and friends. One is that celiac is not well known.[4] A 2022 survey conducted by the Harris Poll on behalf of Beyond Celiac found that half of Americans know nothing about either celiac disease or gluten sensitivity.[5] "When I was first diagnosed," Emma wrote on the celiac.com forum, "my family didn't believe there was such a thing as Celiac Disease. My family actually googled the term to see if I made it up. That hurt a whole lot." Emma continued to get into arguments with family members who insisted she had "a simple food allergy" (October 26, 2008). Arthur's relatives assumed that his pickiness about food stemmed from psychological problems. "My uncle thinks I have OCD and said I need to talk to someone." Arthur's aunt also was skeptical that he had a "real" disease: "Whenever I discuss health issues her response is 'oh please, your grandparents lived to their 90s and you can't worry about this all the time'" (December 2, 2010).

Many people who have heard of celiac disease underestimate its severity and chronic nature. The Beyond Celiac survey reported that just 20 percent of Americans understand that untreated celiac disease can lead to depression and anxiety, 17 percent realize it can lead to neurological disorders, 15 percent realize it can lead to anemia, 12 percent realize it can lead to osteoporosis or osteopenia, 11 percent realize it can lead to some types of cancer, 11 percent realize it can lead to delayed growth in children, and 9 percent realize it can lead to infertility.[6] Forum participants complained about friends and family who did not understand that celiac disease was a lifelong condition. "I'm really at a loss for what to do at the moment," Madison wrote. Because she was sixteen, she still lived with her father, who

> doesn't quite seem to understand that because I'm a celiac, I can't have ANY traces of gluten, and that it's a lifelong commitment, and seems to be in denial that I have the disorder. He's always telling me that he's sure I'll be able to eat anything I want after the damage to my small intestine is healed. . . . No matter how many times I tell him that I can never have anything with gluten in it again when he starts in, he just tells me that he's sure I'll be able to have traces of it without any problems at all. . . . He was a nurse in the Navy and is quite convinced that he's right about the matter because he has more of a medical background than I do (I'm only a nursing assistant.) (August 29, 3006)

June's mother similarly insisted that the disorder would "just go away" (August 26, 2011). The actress Jennifer Esposito wrote about a friend who subscribed to the reigning belief that everyone with enough grit and determination can overcome all afflictions. Esposito thus felt like "an alien in a strange world" when she spent summer weekends at the friend's house in the Hamptons. "It was enjoyable and relaxing to sit by the beach and have a few laughs with friends," Esposito wrote. "But it was difficult, too. This particular friend of mine is a great friend to me, but she really doesn't understand celiac disease. She is a 'pick yourself up and dust yourself off and move on' kind of person, and that's a wonderful thing for her, but I felt as though she was frustrated with me. She tried to hide it, but I could see it."[7]

By contrast with the lack of awareness about celiac, information about the gluten-free diet has spread widely. Many people who believe they know everything important about it fail to understand the extreme measures celiacs must take to stay safe. A college student, June was thankful that her parents cooked gluten-free food when she returned home for the summer. They did not realize, however, how rigorously the dietary rules had to be followed. "We all eat out of the same chip bags and candy jars," June wrote, "and I tell them to make sure to shake the chips or whatever onto the plate rather than putting their hands in it." The previous evening "my mom puts her hand in the chip bag after touching her hamburger bun. She's like, 'well, I didn't touch all the chips,' but that's not the point. The point is she was not careful or mindful and the bag is now contaminated." To add insult to injury, the mother "blamed it on me for having celiac because she said it's hard to remember things like that, but seriously it shouldn't be that hard" (June 10, 2018). Elana considered herself fortunate that her parents and brother were largely "understanding that even a speck of gluten will make me sick." She also sympathized with their refusal to eliminate gluten themselves: "The food within the Hispanic culture is filled with gluten and I don't feel right demanding this huge lifestyle change for me." But she could not accept "being subjected to cross-contamination various times due to their carelessness (mostly my dad)." She concluded, "I am frustrated and angry and honestly fed up because at the end of the day my health is on the line" (June 5, 2017).

Having recently moved into her boyfriend's house, Jane wondered how she could explain to his thirteen-year-old son that she could get sick from a single crumb without sounding like "a total freak" or "a crazy overbearing stepmother." She recently had seen the boy fail "to wash his hands after eating a soft pretzel as he was about to prep dinner." Even after "a big discussion" about the various ways her food could be contaminated, she "witnessed the boy prepare a bagel and immediately unload the dishwasher without washing his hands." She acknowledged that "this sounds like dumb stuff," but celiacs "know it can get us sick, and I've pretty much been getting sick weekly since moving in" (June 6, 2017). Daphne preferred to withdraw from friends rather than try to explain dietary rules that appeared so irrational. "My friends just wonder why I disappear for stretches of time and keep canceling plans," Darlene wrote. "I feel so silly saying, 'Well, I had a crumb of bread and now I'm bed-ridden,' so I usually make up excuses, like—um, I have to work! The flu! A last-minute emergency! Sorry, but can't make it tonight!!" (April 1, 2010).

People who follow a gluten-free diet in the absence of a relevant medical diagnosis may be especially likely to claim expertise without any knowledge of celiac dietary prohibitions. "In our community a 'lot' of people are trying to be gluten free," one forum participant wrote.

> At first I thought this was great. I've been surprised that most of these people, however, haven't given a thought to the risks of cross contamination. I've had people tell me that heating our pans to 450 should be fine because "that would kill anything" (never mind plenty of glutinous baked goods cook that high), ask me why we would replace our bamboo flatware tray (full of crumbs in the little cracks and not dishwasher-washable), and not realize we had to go through our condiments, throw out old spices, get rid of old appliances used with wheat or wood utensils, etc. How do you deal with other gluten-free friends not being as stringent as you? (January 7, 2011)

Other sufferers complain that friends and extended family members assume that avoiding gluten is simply a fashionable practice or an excuse for fussiness.[8] Leah was "dreading" an upcoming family reunion because she anticipated "comments along the lines that it [the diet] is just a fad and I'm being picky" (July 19, 2016). Although Bella was initially relieved to learn she had celiac, she had just begun to realize that she never would have her favorite food again. "What really irks me, though," she wrote," is that when I eat with certain extended family and friends, they make comments about how the diet is a marketing ploy, or a silly fad, or how fifty years ago, no one had celiac" (October 25, 2009). Gluten Dude posted a letter from a woman who encountered cruelty as well as miscomprehension. She wrote that she hates "family get together and holidays because 'my diet' generally manages to become a focal point of verbal abuse—despite my pleas for people to just cook and eat whatever they damn well please. I never expect anyone to accommodate me. With Thanksgiving and Christmas on the horizon, I am already bracing for this year's barrage of attacks and guilt trips." One relative "literally rolls her eyes every time I decline to eat something or suggest that we could modify a recipe (or that I could make a GF version to bring to the event). The eye-rolling gets especially pronounced when I express concerns about really obvious cross-contamination hazards. This condition is difficult enough to live with as it is."[9]

Invitations to join friends and relatives at restaurant thus often present a quandary.[10] Should people with celiac insist that they meet only in places known to take adequate precautions? Should celiacs phone the restaurant ahead of time to make special arrangements? Should they eat before they go and plan to order only a salad or drink? Or should they make excuses and stay home? Sylvia dropped out of her book group because it regularly met at a restaurant she considered unsafe. Jocelyn, the wife of a man in the military, wrote,

> I am a member of the spouses group at our base, and I have had to miss the last three play dates because the women planning them plan them AT FAST FOOD RESTAURANTS. Aside from this being terrible for the health of the kids, there are other options available. They always invite me... and I tell them "sorry guys, it's going to be rough being surrounded by food I am allergic to." I am at a point that I don't even want to be a member anymore because people think I am snotty because I don't go. Why should I go, starve, bring my OWN wine, and constantly be worried about [cross-contamination]? (July 28, 2010)

The prospect of eating at the homes of friends or relatives elicits similar fears. Celiacs can monitor or at least observe food preparation in shared households, but they have virtually no control over meals cooked elsewhere. Heather asked other members of the forum, "If someone tells you its [sic] home made and gluten free—how do u know they know what they're saying is true? Do they fully understand what gluten free means so that it definitely is, i.e., someone could to best of their knowledge have made it gluten free but not know that they contaminated it or that they've used ingredients that they believe is gluten free but mite [*sic*] not be in my eyes" (February 22, 2016). Other remarks suggest that those suspicions often are well founded. Laura had been asked to dinner by close friends who knew she was on a gluten-free diet but nevertheless served soups with "massive amounts of breadcrumbs or very thick crusty bread on top" (September 25, 2021). When Georgina received an invitation to dinner at the home of her husband's boss, she called his wife "in advance to tell her that I had celiac and couldn't eat any bread, pasta, etc. She didn't know much about celiac, and I told her not to go to any trouble, but I just wanted to give her a heads up so that she was not insulted if I couldn't eat all of the food she prepared. Well, at lunch she seemed a bit upset when I told her I couldn't eat her orzo salad, and she said, 'Oh, but I didn't put any gluten in it!' Maybe she didn't realize that orzo was pasta?" (December 17, 2010).

Other writers began eating food before realizing it contained gluten. Mary asked, "How do you get someone to realize how important it is for a celiac to be completely gluten free and take no chances?" She had agreed to attend Thanksgiving at her boyfriend's house "on the condition that we cook completely gluten free." The previous year his mother had "made this really yummy and easy mashed potato casserole with instant mashed potatoes. Since I liked it so much I requested it this year, but of course it needed to be gluten free. I knew this could be done since Betty Crocker makes a very obviously labeled gluten-free boxed potatoes. So we are halfway through dinner and we are all commenting on how wonderful everything tastes when his mother says she didn't check the potato box. Oh and guess what—I got sick" (November 30, 2010). Vivian described what happened when her brother-in-law cooked a stuffed roast for Christmas: "He tells me it's gluten free when he puts it out to eat. I take a slice and took 3–4 bites before realizing there was rice in it." Because she knew he liked Rice a Roni, a brand containing gluten, she questioned the food. "Sure enough, it was Rice a Roni. He tells me 'but it's gluten free.' 'No, I don't think so,' I told him. (I knew it wasn't) So he read the box and said 'oh no! Sorry!'" (December 28, 2016).

Nevertheless, celiacs' withdrawal from social situations does not result solely from the attitudes and actions of others. Despite the anger celiacs express toward individuals who ridicule or refuse to cater to their needs, some comments suggest they are ambivalent about asking for accommodations. Viewing themselves as annoyances or "inconveniences," they hesitate to make demands.[11] "The biggest reason I feel so down," Josh wrote after learning he had celiac, "is that I will now be that guy who inconveniences everyone when going out to a restaurant" (July 14, 2020). Sophie commented that her diagnosis "makes me sad because I know it means that it will be an inconvenience to my extended family and friends when we gather for meals or want to go out for dinner" (June 1, 2016). Frances wrote that she probably would be "heading up north to Virginia to spend Christmas/New Years with someone important. Neither he nor his family eat gluten free and I unfortunately have celiac disease. How can I cope while I'm living with them? What can I eat, how should I eat, will I have to prepare every meal I eat by myself? I'm sure we've all felt that we've never wanted to inconvenience anyone" (November 9, 2016).

Having internalized derogatory views about individuals who impose on others, some celiacs express guilt and shame as well as gratitude when they receive accommodations. Jacob asked, "Does anyone ever feel guilty for other people having to accommodate their food needs? We're having a party at work and my coworkers are going out of their way to get gluten free food options but I feel so bad that they went through so much trouble to accommodate my needs. Am I just crazy? Does this get any better with time?" (April 11, 2014). Richard had just spent his first Thanksgiving with his fiancée's family. "VERY LUCKY," he wrote, "that they were willing to prepare an entirely gluten-free meal, use new kitchen utensils and cutting boards, etc." Nevertheless, his pleasure was not unalloyed: "I couldn't help but feel horrible the entire weekend. I feel guilty that I caused them to do these things and take precautions and also felt incredibly singled out all weekend." He, too, viewed himself as a bother. "How do you all deal with emotions related to feeling singled out/like an inconvenience?" he asked (November 29, 2021). Believing himself still to be "on show," Richard may have been especially anxious not to impose on others and appear weak and needy.

Other celiacs may not feel entitled to make claims because they have long disdained people who appear excessively preoccupied with their food. Joanne acknowledged that she used to sneer at anyone she witnessed reading food labels. "Now I'm one of the people I always laughed at," she wrote. "I'm living the life of someone I never wanted to have to deal with. I always became so annoyed by my mom and aunt constantly talking about nutrition and talking Paleo and all the other diet fads. Little did I know, I would become one" (February 15, 2015). Embodying the characteristics she once considered demeaning, Joanne refrained from asking for special treatment.

In addition, many celiacs want to avoid offending members of their social network who offer food as a sign of affection or view cooking as a craft and expect appreciation for their skills. Selma noted that her relatives "do most things homemade and if you don't eat, feelings are generally hurt" (April 21, 2014). Marianne referred to "all the relatives and friends not understanding why I would refuse to eat bread, cakes, etc. and sometimes taking it as a personal insult if I do not try their cooking" (April 6, 2014). Justine had waited for three years after her diagnosis to feel comfortable enough to attend a party in a house that was not gluten free. "Now I understand what all of you were talking about when you shared your party stories," she wrote. "The host, my friend who knows about my food limitations, couldn't understand when I turned down everything she offered me. She was even surprised when I didn't want a piece of her homemade cake that had several things in it that I don't eat—gluten/grains, dairy, eggs, sugar, etc. She seemed hurt that I couldn't enjoy something special she had made, it was hard to disappoint her" (March 15, 2015). Harper discovered that even bringing her own food could cause distress. The host was uncomfortable seeing me not eating or drinking anything, so I took out the water and food I brought. Then people were upset that I was eating out of plastic baggies. It didn't bother me. I was surprised that everyone was so concerned, I'm so used to eating with no frills. Next time I'll bring my food in containers or put it on a plate before I eat it, so the others will feel more convinced that I'm enjoying myself. Or if anyone has suggestions on how I can blend in better next time, and not stand out so much, I'd love to hear them. (March 15, 2015)

"Passing" represents the most extreme form of blending in. One commentator describes passing "as a form of imposture in which members of a marginalized group presented themselves as members of a dominant group. African Americans passing for white, for example, or Jews passing for gentiles, were attempting to achieve the appearance of equality or to neutralize the stigma of those racialized and religious identities."[12] Questions about revealing a celiac diagnosis loom especially large in two settings. One is dating. The search for a romantic partner forces everyone with a disability to confront the issue of disclosure in an especially intense way.[13] Unlike those with visible disabilities, people diagnosed with celiac can exercise some discretion about when to divulge personal health information. Because dating often involves eating in restaurants, however, celiacs have to decide how much to reveal sooner than other people with invisible disabilities. More than two-thirds of the participants in a Columbia University study reported that celiac disease had a "major" or "moderate" impact on their experience dating. Thirty-eight percent of the respondents said that they were uncomfortable explaining their needs to restaurant waiters, 28 percent took risks while eating out, and 8 percent intentionally ate food containing gluten.[14]

Actress Jennifer Esposito recommends

> knowing someone pretty well and trusting them before you give them too much of your personal history. If you give people too much, then the questions come rolling out, and they may be questions you don't want to

answer, or comments that will sting. I think I've heard them all. That I don't eat because I'm on a diet, or I want to stay skinny, or I'm vain. That I don't eat this or that, so I must not know how to have fun. That I should just eat the topping of the pizza or scrape the breading off the chicken.[15]

But some forum writers feared that they would be forced to reveal too much health information prematurely. "I've been gluten-free for almost a year now," Jasper wrote, "and am starting to feel better somewhat. I didn't bother dating while I was going through the healing process because I was just too sick. Now that my health has improved some I'd like to start dating again, but it always ends up with my trying to explain that I can't eat out and it gets awkward and the date doesn't happen or goes badly because I have yet to find someone who understands celiac" (September 20, 2016). Nicholas was recently divorced. "I'm ready to get back out and start dating again," he commented, "but it is hard. I have no trouble talking to people and getting dates but then dinner comes up or snacks at the movies or drinks at a bar. Celiac disease is probably my biggest challenge ever and it's asking a lot to ask someone to understand" (November 27, 2016). Believing that her relationship had progressed to the point of a first kiss, Julia wondered how she could explain her need for caution. "I've heard about being potentially glutened via a kiss," she explained. "How do I broach this? I don't want to scare him off or make him think that I'm a lot of hard work. I know he's going to have to accept me as I am, etc., but for someone new to the entire thing, it is likely overwhelming. . . . He's a lovely guy so I do think he'll be understanding, but if anyone has any advice of first hand experience on how to approach this topic without it being a weird moment, that would be great" (June 29, 2016).

Work

The issue of disclosure also frequently emerges in the workplace, where projecting an image of strength and competence is especially critical.

Two sociologists quoted a woman who insisted that her husband made no attempt to hide his diagnosis. Because he often traveled for work, "he's always eating with people and he's up there and saying I can't have this and people think he is a jerk because (laughs) they don't know it is very serious. He is brazen about it; really gets in their face . . . he is very open about it, he can't hide it. If anyone crosses him, boy, he lets them know."[16] Although we do not learn what position this man occupied, we can assume he enjoyed considerable power and prestige. The same researchers quoted a woman who felt insecure about her job. Having recently been hired by a large law firm, she occasionally endangered her health by eating unsafe food to conceal her condition: "In my line of work we host clients for lunch all the time. I can't just sit there and not eat. I don't want to shift the focus to my problem and seem weak . . . like I can't handle it. I have to do what I need in order to work, especially in this economy."[17]

Writing on the celiac.com forum, Laura explained why she feared that revealing her diagnosis would undermine her employment prospects: "This is my first, ever, real job. And these people are super picky about who they hire. And I'm scared that if I tell them about my issues, they're not going to want to rehire me in the spring (I'm a seasonal employee) because it'll qualify me as high maintenance" (August 17, 2007). Although Laura does not explain what she meant by "high maintenance," we can assume she worried that employers would consider her an undesirable job candidate because she might increase their insurance burden, take too many sick days, or have difficulty fulfilling her responsibilities,

Passing, however, frequently exacts a toll. Robin had just learned that her forthcoming interview for a job she "really" wanted would involve lunch. "I have no idea what to expect," she wrote, "but I'm sure it won't be easy to negotiate. All the etiquette advice I read online said, 'Don't make a big deal when you're dining at an interview.' I value my health greatly, but I also don't want to be remembered as the chick who made such a big deal about the croutons!" (June 21, 2005). Rose also worried about exposure. "My immediate boss and coworkers know about my celiac," she wrote, "but company doesn't, and I expect to keep it that way." She had just learned she was required to attend a day-long conference where lunch would be served. "I am doomed," she concluded (September 8, 2013). Frank was "trying to fly under the radar with my health issues" because he was on a six-month trial period. "I did not reveal to my employer that I have celiac disease," he wrote. "Although I am good at my job, it would be perceived as weakness and possible 'trouble' for my employer. Thus far, I have showed that I am a hard worker always coming early or on time to work and diligently doing my duties." But he faced a dilemma: "Taking any time off to go to a doctor will raise other questions and possibly negatively affect my employment." He had a forthcoming doctor's appointment that would require him to arrive at work late. "I would definitely make sure that I stay longer at work and make up for the missed time at work," he continued. "But I am not sure how to explain being late 2 hours. How can I tell them that I had to go to a doctor? If I do say I needed to see a doctor, should I downplay it (and if so, how) so that they do not ask other questions or require me to provide a detailed dr's note since the note would state what and why they were doing these tests? I hate that I cannot just be honest" (February 2, 2015).

Regardless of whether or not celiacs reveal their diagnoses at work, various symptoms can hamper their productivity. Sy wrote that he had "all sorts of manifestations" from celiac. "One in particular is peripheral neuropathic pain shooting down my left arm and into my left hand. It hurts quite a bit quite often, and other times, when more relaxed, goes into a numb state. So it makes it a little difficult to be on the computer for long periods of time, which 95% of my job requires in the technology field" (March 31, 2013). Harold was so tired that he decided to take Adderall, an amphetamine, to help him do his job. When he had a bad reaction, he decided he was "done with drugs. Forever." He worried, however, that "I won't be able to be productive at work. I know I should eat well, take supplements, and exercise. But even with all that I can't focus and fall asleep[.] I've been dx'd [diagnosed] with celiac for over a year and a half, but I can't beat the fatigue" (October 23, 2013). Elaine "had a ton of work to do but unfortunately the brain fog and body aches are not helping" (October 10, 2016).

Many celiacs who disclose their diagnosis discover that honesty may not be the best policy. Like the family and friends discussed earlier in this chapter, most bosses know little about the disease. Judith's employer was suspicious of her request for accommodations because he doubted that celiac was a legitimate disease, as serious as other conditions. "My boss told me that the time I took off feeling ill and seeing doctors was unjustified," Judith wrote, "because I ended up not having a 'real' illness, like cancer or something." As a result, any absence "would have to come out of vacation and not sick time" (June 21, 2015). Viewing the gluten-free diet as a fad, Don's employer joined Don's work colleagues in ridiculing his refusal to eat the bagels and pizza someone brought to the office. Janine tried to explain to her boss that she experiences "unbelievable" pain, nausea, and loss of sleep, among other symptoms, when she gets glutened and worried about driving in that condition. The boss responded, "Sometimes I don't feel good and don't get a lot of sleep, but I still get up early and do what I have to do because I'm the only one who can do it" (December 17, 2009). Larry, a pharmacist who traveled between hospitals in remote areas of Arizona, wrote, "The agency I work for wants me to work 40 hrs. a week and drive 600 miles a week to work at a clinic. When I try to explain that after a 30 day stint it takes a whole day just to get enough energy to take a walk, they don't get it." He added, "They make me feel like such a malingerer" (May 7, 2007).

Other bosses fail to comprehend the enormous amount of energy celiacs must devote to deciding what they can eat. Adam had volunteered for a field trip but asked to be excused when he learned it would involve lunch at an Italian restaurant. "I have been sick a lot of the time lately," he explained, "because, aside from needing to avoid gluten, I have a lot of other food intolerances because my gut is so sensitive—to mushrooms, onions, peppers, etc. Plus, going to an Italian restaurant I don't know with tons of possibilities of wheat contamination is so not worth the risk, it's ridiculous." Nevertheless, when he tried to back out, his boss, "actually got visibly angry and said, 'Well, I think it's really silly for you not to go for such a reason.'" Adam regarded that response as "beyond insensitive, trying to make me feel like a criminal or a bad employee for trying to protect my health" (October 5, 2010). Amy had hoped her boss would understand that spontaneity was not an option when it came to food. When she told him that she had to carefully plan her meals before she traveled with him for a day, he responded that she need not worry because they would "just pick [up] something on the fly." "I am not okay with this," she stressed. "What do I do? Freaking out!" (May 27, 2015).

Cynthia's bosses assumed that celiac was a short-term condition she could easily overcome if she put her mind to it. She had worked at a family firm for years when she became ill and learned she had celiac. A "verbally abusive" CEO ran the company with his two nephews. "After a violent outburst from the CEO," she wrote, "I asked one of the nephews why they won't support me, and this was his reply: 'All three of us resent you because you have missed so much over the last two years, and we just don't think that you want to be here.' He thinks that I should just clean all of the gluten out of my system and then I will be fine" (October 2, 2005).

Several participants reported fear of reprisals. Julie wondered if any other forum participant faced her predicament: "When I 'get glutened' and become sick, the symptoms can last for a while (and even come and go without warning). One day, it's doable and the next, it's not. On the not-so-doable days, I have had to call out of work. Nobody wants to be in a bunch of pain and/or going to the bathroom a bunch during work. I got in trouble the other day for calling out, though, which was quite frustrating" (April 30, 2014). A certified nurse assistant, Nadine wrote that she "had to call in a lot because I either can't drive or I'm afraid to pass out at work. I'm so afraid of getting fired and I need money to pay my bills" (April 1, 2016). Sonia understood that she was on borrowed time. She had been at the same job for nearly eleven years, but in the three years before her diagnosis, she wrote, "brain fog and lack of focus caused huge problems with my ability to do my job properly." Soon after inaugurating a gluten-free diet, her "job performance improved and things got better and better." But then, three months before writing, she "noticed a decline happening, along with some almost constant glutening symptoms." Now she was beginning to improve again, but she still made mistakes, and her boss had just told her that after one more mistake she would be "out." Sonia understood his position: he had been patient for many years but he had a company to run and needed to be able to count on his employees. She was "terrified, though, because there are no other jobs in my area that I'm qualified for and I have no back-up plan" (June 24, 2008).

Celiacs who receive accommodations worry about exhausting their employers' benevolence. Jerome wrote,

> I have been gluten free now for 3 months and yet I feel like at least once every 2 weeks I am calling in sick. Waking up in the morning I never know if I am going to be going into work or not [because] I don't know how I am going to feel. I know everyone and my doctors have said the first 6 months to a year are the worst and things should get better—that's great I am looking forward to that BUT how do I tell my boss that? I have used all my sick/vacation time and I just don't know how much longer people might be understanding about my call ins. (August 26, 2014)

A month into his new diet, Jacob was "battling with low energy, muscle weakness, ab discomfort, and hours-long headaches" and "feeling like I am unable to keep up with the work-load at my job, even though the working hours (at my doctor's request) have already been cut back." Unfortunately, he continued, "my employer is becoming less and less sympathetic with each passing week, because she is faced with staffing shortages and is pressuring me to work more hours." Jacob's other concern was that his reputation among his office mates would suffer: "I'm feeling like a wimp, and beginning to feel like others think I am faking all these symptoms (which I'm NOT!)" (March 23, 2010).

The relationship between work and symptoms can go both ways. If some symptoms hinder the ability to work, some working conditions trigger or exacerbate symptoms. The forum participants viewed two occupations as especially risky. One was working in a bakery. Mark had recently been diagnosed with celiac. He was loath to leave his job because he was a "specialty dessert and cake decorator" with "an outstanding amount of clients that keep me busy and have me booked far into the next few years." He asked, "Can I still work with flour everyday? I am really hoping the answer is yes even if I have to wear a mask." The forum moderator did not answer the question but warned about "gluten finding its way into your gut through inhalation of wheat flour dust" (August 9, 2022).

Caring for small children was another. "I need help!" Joan began. "I just started working as a nanny 2 weeks ago and I've been consistently glutened from the toddlers I work with. One is 1.5, the other is 2.4 years. So for all of you with babies, you know how messy it is all day. I'm constantly covered in crackers, cereal bars, snack stuff. It's a gluten nightmare" (February 14, 2010). The children Caitlyn taught were slightly older (four and five), but she faced a similar challenge. She was thankful that her reactions to cross-contamination were "not as violent as some people's descriptions," but she "got really tired," had "headaches and brain fog, joint pain, and digestive ick," and became "cranky and depressed." Because she had both a three- and a five-year-old at home, she had made her house gluten free, but she could not do the same in her classroom: "The kids eat lunch there. And snack. And this year breakfast is available in the classroom as well." Although Caitlyn cleaned the tables, swept the floor, and washed her hands regularly, she had recently become sick. "Is this a hopeless situation?" she asked (September 3, 2011).

Other workers also feared contamination. Francesca complained that her coworkers "won't clean up after themselves at the office so our little kitchen area is inches deep in crumbs. . . . Every day there are bagels, coffee cakes, desserts, cookies, sandwiches—whatever—sitting around.

There is NO clean place and if there is a clean place it will be dirty before the end of the day. Right now I try to make my food at my desk except when I have to use the microwave (which is most days)" (May 9, 2007). Penelope worked for a company that provided services to factories throughout the country. Her job required her to travel to different locations. She wrote just after she had been working at a flour mill, "Obviously I am exposed to gluten at this mill. I was inside their offices and in our work trailer on the site. In plain view from our trailer is a car that looks like it is coated in dough." Although she tried to explain her predicament to her boss, she could not determine where she was sent. "The main problem," she continued, "is that I have no skills that are in demand. I cannot just quit my job. I have nothing, no savings, no family, absolutely nothing that can be used to support me, other than to continue at this job" (Penelope, 2012). Terry's job description at a car rental business required him to clean cars. "Picture a minivan with crackers all smooshed in the seats and on the floor," he wrote. "I wear gloves but how many times a day do you think I touch my face? I lick my lips, scratch my lips. It is very hard for me to do this cause I feel like there is so much [cross-contamination] in rental cars" (December 30, 2007). Gloria could exercise control over her classroom but only when she was there. Every Friday she moved to a different room while another teacher sat at her desk. "Today I walk in," Gloria wrote, "and the teacher is eating from a bag of crackers at my desk and has cracker crumbs on it. I stopped in my tracks." After Gloria explained the situation, the other teacher agreed to be more careful in the future. But Gloria wondered if she "could ever feel safe anywhere" (October 1, 2010).

Several other forum participants discussed the difficulties of managing diarrhea at work. One of the few forum participants in a blue-collar job, Dennis worked at a machine shop. "I was getting reprimanded for being in the bathroom too much," he wrote, "even after I have told them I have been confirmed as having Celiac's disease, and they have no bathroom policy. I feel like because they don't have it or understand they think I am making up the fact that if I eat something that bothers my stomach,

I end up with a green light from my stomach to the end of the line all day. It's gone as far as me getting in shouting matches with my foreman" (September 24, 2009). Rachel worked at a climbing gym. She often had diarrhea, but the only restroom was "outside, WAY at the end of the soccer field.... I have to actually lock up and can really only go when there are no customers" (February 26, 2006). A cashier, Sadie had no one to fill in for her when she had to run to the bathroom (August 17, 2007).

Several forum participants in professional and managerial positions had to travel for business or attend conferences and retreats. Those created additional problems. Elsa was grateful that her office had made reservations for her at a Chicago hotel. But when she called ahead, the "conversation did not go well." She elaborated:

> The coordinator said they were "very well acquainted" with celiac disease. Ha! She said that surely I would be able to find some safe things on the buffet. I said I did not feel comfortable with that as the risk of [cross-contamination] is too high and I'm ridiculously sensitive to gluten, dairy, and soy. She seemed very put off by this and said maybe the chef would make me a separate meal. I asked about their cooking methods—do they have a separate prep surface, or separate place on the grill? No. Well, could they use a separate pan to make my food please? No. She said they're "too small of a hotel to be able to do that kind of thing." All cooking surfaces, even pans, are shared with all ingredients.

Elsa added, "I'm freaking out here—I have to fly in so it's not like I can bring 3 days worth of food. And I won't have a car to go buy any. What on earth do I do?" (October 25, 2010). At least once a month Carmela traveled to "a very rural area," where her options were limited to "fast food and Applebees or the local pizza, Chinese and Mexican place" (March 24, 2013). Arleen soon would attend her first out-of-town conference since her diagnosis. "It's being catered in," she wrote, "and there won't be an opportunity to leave to get food or to have access to a fridge and microwave. I may just tell them not to worry about it and bring rice cakes and peanut butter. I'm dreading it" (February 5, 2014). Lara's "big worry" was a two-day retreat with "a big dinner on the first night" at "some kind of barbecue place" that was unlikely to have food she could eat (July 14, 2013).

Having mastered many of the intricacies of working in sales at his company while living with celiac, Jeremy worried that he was locked into a position he yearned to escape. He explained his dilemma this way:

> I can still remember how terrified I was when I started and constantly feared how I would handle eating while on the road. Now I don't even think twice, but I am considering taking a new job with another company and am afraid of having to deal with all the stuff I dealt with at my current job when I first started—the awkwardness at company dinners, having to explain over and over again to people the whole gluten thing and having people bust my balls about it. That alone is incentive enough to never leave my company, but I want to advance myself and make more $. (April 29, 2010)

A number of forum participants left the labor force, at least temporarily. Those included a lawyer, a teacher, and the head cook in a nursing home. Valerie wrote that she "worked in a very stressful environment for 3 ½ years. Well during this time is when I began getting sick; we all know how bosses are, every time I was out sick (which was not that often) I would hear about it. I went to work for over a year in constant pain! I finally decided to quit last September" (March 5, 2004). Maya also experienced pain. A single mother, she had been unemployed for most of the time since her daughter was born, three years earlier. "I am really wanting to work and make a better life for us," she wrote, "but how am I supposed to keep a job with this problem?" (March 5, 2004). Some of those who returned to the labor force tried to work part-time, thus forfeiting some of their salary, or at home.

Yet other celiacs were horrified to discover their chosen careers were now closed to them. The military disqualifies people with celiac from service because Meals Ready-to-Eat (MREs) do not have gluten-free options.[18] "My whole life I've been dreaming about the day that I could join the National Guard!" Janice exclaimed. "It has been something that I never had to think about wanting to do. Well I'm finally old enough to join which is the best thing ever! But—I have celiac. My recruiter has informed me that because of my allergy I can't go through with my dream. I have spent many nights crying about this. I no longer know what to do with my life" (November 18, 2015). Chris used similar language: joining the military had "always been a dream of mine and now I've been told it can disqualify me. It was always good to know I could join but now knowing I can't ever it just really sucks not being able to follow a long time dream of mine" (December 1, 2016).

John feared he would meet a similar disappointment in law enforcement: "I never thought having Celiac would stop me from advancing in my career and in my life. Sadly I might not get hired for a job in law enforcement because they state, 'Symptoms and signs of organic upper digestive tract disease may be disqualifying.' . . . I'm tired of being broke in a job I can't bear to continue" (May 27, 2014).

Conclusion

Paraphrasing Heinz Kohut, two researchers write that "people seek to confirm a subjective sense of belongingness or 'being part of' in order to avoid feelings of loneliness and alienation."[19] Many celiacs, however, feel socially disconnected. Because the strictures of the dietary prohibitions flout common sense, family and friends view celiacs' refusal to eat certain food as characterological flaws rather than medical necessities. Without the accommodations that would enable them to stay safe, celiacs often are excluded, or exclude themselves, from the various social events that center on food.

Because certain foods are central to the sense of belonging to some ethnic and religious communities, celiacs from those groups are especially likely to feel like outsiders when they are forced to restrict their diets. Previous chapters included two examples. One was a man who wrote that his celiac diagnosis was difficult for him because he was "of Italian heritage and now my nonna can't cook all the things she used to for me." He felt upset thinking about how his diet would affect "relationships with those close to me" (July 14, 2020). The other, a woman, explained her inability to stop eating gluten this way: "I am Mexican and food is a central part of our life and family traditions." Eliminating gluten might challenge her sense of ethnic identity and undermine intimate ties. Here we heard from Elana, who refrained from asking her family to give up gluten because "the food within the Hispanic culture is filled with gluten and I don't feel right demanding this huge lifestyle change for me."

The few studies that examine the labor-force participation of people with celiac find that they experience significantly more work loss than their counterparts.[20] This chapter can help us understand why. In some cases, disease symptoms hinder workers' ability to fulfill their responsibilities; in others, employment conditions trigger or worsen symptoms. Moreover, although employees with disabilities can request reasonable accommodations from their employers under the Rehabilitation Act of 1973, the Americans with Disabilities Act (ADA) of 1990, and the ADA Amendments Act of 2009, celiacs rarely receive special treatment at work. We heard little from blue-collar workers, who undoubtedly encounter the most serious problems contending with celiac symptoms on the job, but the white-collar employees participating on the celiac.com forum found few bosses willing to respond to their needs.

Conclusion

The diverse meanings of the word "access" provide a starting point for reviewing this book's major themes. Celiacs confront issues of access in the context of both medicine and disability. Ronald M. Andersen, a major researcher in the field of healthcare access, defines the concept as "the actual use of personal health services and everything that facilitates or impedes the use of personal health services."[1] Two of the measures Andersen proposes for the effectiveness of healthcare access are "promoting early detection and diagnosis" and "reducing the effects of chronic disease."[2] Celiac disease care does not fare well according to either metric.

Researchers report that approximately half of all people with celiac remain undiagnosed and that most of those who receive diagnoses have waited for them for years. The personal accounts we read highlight the many physical and emotional problems celiacs experience during the long interval between presenting symptoms and obtaining a label for them. Many people report going from doctor to doctor to try to understand the cause of their suffering. Some obtain psychiatric diagnoses that infuriate them. In the absence of timely and accurate diagnoses, celiacs are unable to take appropriate treatment and thus remain at high risk of several diseases that can shorten life.

Andersen notes that one indicator of the second measure is the number of physician contacts.[3] Although the American College of Gastroenterology recommends that patients visit doctors regularly after diagnosis, that advice rarely is honored.[4] In many cases, however, the cause lies not in barriers to care but rather in the widespread and well-founded belief that doctors have little to offer. Numerous studies have documented the growing distrust of medical expertise among the general population.[5]

Celiacs whose diagnoses were delayed for years or whose physicians failed to offer advice about managing the disorder may be especially likely to lose faith in the medical profession. We know much less about contacts with dieticians and nutritionists, two professionals who should have a major role in celiac care, but it is clear that both inadequate insurance coverage for their visits and widespread skepticism about their value deter many celiacs from consulting them. The lack of professional oversight leaves celiacs especially vulnerable to the enticements and promises of social media influencers and food industry marketers.

It has become almost a cliché to state that food is medicine in celiac care. Examining access to gluten-free food is thus more critical than exploring access to health care. Poverty and residence in food deserts, commonly cited as major factors in reducing food access, are especially significant for people with celiac. Because gluten-free products are more expensive than their wheat counterparts, they deplete low food budgets more rapidly. Many poor people can find work only in the contingent labor force, which leaves little time for home cooking. Food banks provide few items that celiacs can eat. And without access to supermarkets, people are relegated to convenience stores and fast-food restaurants that rarely stock gluten-free products. A disproportionate number of food-insecure people are members of racially marginalized groups.[6] Researchers estimate that one-sixth of Americans with celiac, or five hundred thousand people, are food insecure.[7]

The impact of residence in long-term institutions on access to gluten-free food demands greater attention. Researchers have looked primarily at the problems of college and university students whose education suffers when they cannot find gluten-free items on campus. The little available information about nursing homes and assisted living facilities suggests that those institutions frequently deny admission to celiacs and refuse to cater to the dietary needs of those who enroll. The twenty-two million incarcerated Americans have little access to healthy food of any kind. Adherence to the gluten-free diet is virtually impossible for the overwhelming majority of those with celiac.

The social model of disability shifts the emphasis from individual impairments to the surrounding environment, asking not how we can correct or improve disabled bodies but rather how we can promote social, economic, and political participation. After focusing almost exclusively on physical access to public buildings and transportation for many years, disability scholars have begun to give greater prominence to a broader set of barriers to social integration, including intangible ones.[8] Two major obstacles celiacs face are the widespread disparagement of anyone on a gluten-free diet and the lack of awareness of the disease. Because the gluten-free diet is commonly viewed as a lifestyle choice made by privileged members of society, celiacs often encounter derision and disbelief when they insist that they must avoid gluten. Forum participants complained of being told that a gluten-free diet was a "marketing ploy" or "a silly fad."

Not only do friends and family mock all gluten-free diets; they also fail to understand the rigor of the celiac dietary regimen and the severe consequences of deviating from it. As a result, members of celiacs' social networks belittle their complaints and refuse to accommodate them. As we saw in the previous chapter, a woman wrote to Gluten Dude that one relative "literally rolls her eyes every time I decline to eat something or suggest that we could modify a recipe. . . . The eye rolling gets especially pronounced when I express concerns about really obvious cross-contamination hazards." The lack of observable symptoms compounds the difficulty. Although some celiacs want to "pass" as healthy, others believe their needs are more easily discounted because they do not look sick. Employers accuse celiacs with repeated absences of being deliberately deceitful or "malingerers," exploiting physical limitations to win exemption from work. Members of shared households fail to observe basic celiac precautions. Friends and families become offended when celiacs reject invitations to dine at their houses or join gatherings at restaurants.

But we also have seen that many celiacs are ambivalent about asking for special consideration because they share the common American belief that dependence of any kind demonstrates personal inadequacy. We recall one man who expressed guilt and embarrassment, not just gratitude, when his fiancée's family prepared a separate Thanksgiving meal for him. Several forum participants noted that they were reluctant to "inconvenience" others. Some also were determined not to discomfort those who view any kind of disability with distaste. A woman wanted to know how she could make others feel at ease when she ate her own food at a social gathering.

The pervasiveness of the ideology of personal responsibility also may inhibit celiacs from making claims. Just as many people believe that the government should not pay for the medical care of skiers who break their legs on slopes, smokers who are diagnosed with lung cancer, and all those who suffer from problems associated with obesity, so many celiacs assume they should be able to detect and avoid all the hazards surrounding them. Some forum participants expressed rage when food labels were confusing or misleading and restaurants servers failed to respect orders for gluten-free meals. Others, however, presumed a level of personal control that contrasted with the reality of their lives; as a result, they placed the blame on themselves rather than on improper labeling or a restaurant's negligence.

It is possible, of course, that some of those glutened in restaurants had relaxed their guard because they were away from home. "I feel like when I go out to eat I am in denial I have celiac," one forum participant wrote. "I don't purposely eat [gluten]. I just assume some things are ok, when they're not" (September 17, 2016). Abigail Carroll notes that Americans view eating out as a gift to themselves. "When we treat ourselves to a meal at a restaurant," she comments, "we do not skimp because skimping would defeat the purpose." The large amount of alcohol consumed in restaurants also encourages indulgence.[9] But celiacs who hold themselves responsible for all gluten exposure in restaurants ignore the obligation of those establishments (especially the ones representing food as gluten free) to train their staff well, establish safe kitchen practices for cross-contamination, and ensure they are rigorously followed.

Nevertheless, celiacs engage in various forms of activism. They have signed petitions and written letters to protest derisive comments and jokes in the media about the gluten-free diet. After joining forces with allergy groups to pass the Food Allergen Labeling and Consumer Protection Act (FALCPA), celiac advocates spearheaded a drive to compel the FDA to establish standards for products labeled gluten free. More recently, the Gluten Free Watchdog launched a campaign demanding that the agency enforce its ruling. And all the major celiac organizations repeatedly press members of Congress to pass legislation expanding FALCPA's provisions, regulating gluten-free claims in restaurants, and restricting gluten in medications.

Despite the impressive achievements of those organizations in helping celiacs manage their disease and advocating on their behalf, this book has raised questions about the extent to which corporate funding distorts the agendas of some of those groups. The most urgent issue celiacs face is obtaining healthy, gluten-free food, but four organizations solicit financial contributions from companies that produce expensive, ultraprocessed, high-caloric items. The Celiac Disease Foundation (CDF) follows physicians and dietitians in advising celiacs to choose whole foods that are naturally free of gluten; its website, however, is replete with advertisements from industry sponsors that overwhelm that message. The CDF also receives criticism for its failure to mention expert advice about Cheerios, the breakfast cereal made with gluten-free sorted oats, that is produced by one of its major funders.

Partnerships with the pharmaceutical industry may help explain why advocacy organizations argue that it is essential to develop a drug therapy to eliminate the need to adhere to a gluten-free diet. I have noted repeatedly that although all celiacs can benefit from a pill that would eliminate the consequences of inadvertent gluten exposure, promises of a drug treatment that would eradicate celiac are unlikely to be fulfilled in the near future. Most pharmaceutical therapies will be effective only in conjunction with the gluten-free diet. Here we might add that it is unlikely that any kind of drug will appear as quickly as celiacs have been led to believe. On May 12, 2022, the Columbia University Irving Medical Center announced, "Drugs for Celiac Disease May Be on the Horizon." The article quoted Benjamin Lebwohl, director of clinical research at the Celiac Disease Center at Columbia University and an associate professor of medicine at the Vagelos College of Physicians and Surgeons, who "felt optimistic that clinical trials could lead to the approval of at least one of [the dozens of] candidate drugs within the next decade."[10] But one month later the single celiac drug in a phase 3 trial was discontinued.[11] Members of the diabetes community complain that they are told over and over that "the cure is five years away."[12] Celiacs similarly may begin to wonder why they must continue to wait for a therapy they repeatedly have been promised.

Researchers in other fields have begun to acknowledge that the emphasis on breakthrough treatments has diverted attention from social and political reforms needed to improve sufferers' lives now. Thomas P. Insel described the moment when he realized that he wrongly may have prioritized genetic research as director of the National Institute of Mental Health. He had been lecturing advocates about scientific successes when he saw a man in the audience becoming increasingly agitated. Taking the microphone, the man said, "'You really don't get it. My 23-year-old son has schizophrenia. He has been hospitalized five times, made three suicide attempts, and now he is homeless. Our house is on fire and you are talking about the chemistry of the paint.'" Although Insel's first response was to defend the research he had promoted for many years, he quickly recognized the "disconnect between the work that I was doing supporting brilliant scientists and dedicated clinicians and the challenges that faced more than 14 million Americans living, and dying, with serious mental illness." He resolved to devote greater attention to expanding and improving patient care.[13] Some Alzheimer's disease researchers have recommended that at least some resources now devoted to clinical drug trials should be shifted to social services.[14]

Medical history is littered with examples of remedies that initially were hailed as miracle cures but failed to deliver on their promise. Some impediments arise from social and cultural circumstances. In his classic 1985 book *No Magic Bullet*, historian Allan M. Brandt asked why, although drug treatments had successfully combated many lethal infectious illnesses, venereal disease remained uncontrolled for many years. The answer, he discovered, lay in the stigma attached to that affliction.[15] More recently, medical historian Erica Charters reminds us that epidemics "do not have the sort of neat, objective endings we may imagine. A swift and decisive endpoint, achieved through the speedy application of scientific innovation—a magic bullet treatment—is usually wishful thinking." Although many of us assumed that the arrival of a COVID-19 vaccine would signal the end of the pandemic, it lingered as a result of government ineptitude, inequitable access to health care, and widespread distrust of all vaccines.[16] In addition, some therapies prove to be less effective than expected. Cochlear implants can improve the ability of deaf people to receive audio information but cannot fully restore hearing; moreover, some people receive no benefits from them.[17]

And some treatments create new problems. The 1921 discovery of insulin dramatically extended the lives of diabetic sufferers, but they soon faced a new set of devastating symptoms. As historian and physician Chris Feudtner writes, "Insulin has not been a panacea."[18] The recent, dramatic increase in its price has placed insulin out of reach for many people who need it. People who have received organ transplants tell us that although they welcome the new lease on life, the side effects of immunosuppression drugs can be brutal.[19] The announcement in January 2023 that a gene therapy to cure sickle cell anemia might soon be approved by the Food and Drug Administration engendered fears that only the wealthy would be able to afford it; some sufferers also worried about how they would fare when the disease no longer dominates their lives.[20] The chemotherapy and radiation that forestall the death of many people with cancer have left some with a raft of serious disabilities.[21] If we emphasize the social, political, and economic factors that hinder adherence to a gluten-free diet, we can direct more attention to remedies that may do far more than pills to relieve the burdens of life with celiac disease, even if they do not increase investor profits.

ACKNOWLEDGMENTS

I received extremely helpful comments from Margaret K. Nelson, Janet Farrell Brodie, Richard Abel, and Laura Abel, who read the entire manuscript, and from Carla Bittel, Charlotte Borst, Sharla Fett, Nina Gelbart, Janet Golden, Heather Abel, and Alice Wexler, who read selected chapters. Daniel Fernandez did excellent research on the major celiac advocacy organizations. At NYU Press, Ilene Kalish once again provided useful comments and essential support, Alexia Traganas shepherded the manuscript through the production process, and Emily Wright did meticulous copy editing. The first chapter is a revised version of my article "The Rise and Fall of Celiac Disease in the United States," *Journal of the History of Medicine and Allied Sciences* 65, no. 1 (January 2010): 71–105. The journal is published by Oxford University Press. Above all, I thank my children and grandchildren, who have learned to live beyond celiac and taught me most of what I know about the disease.

NOTES

INTRODUCTION

1. Benjamin Lebwohl and Alberto Rubio-Tapia, "Epidemiology, Presentation, and Diagnosis of Celiac Disease," *Gastroenterology* 160, no. 1 (January 2021): 63–75; James King et al., "Incidence of Celiac Disease Is Increasing over Time: A Systematic Review and Meta-analysis," *American Journal of Gastroenterology* 115, no. 5 (April 2020): 507–25.
2. Although the word "celiacs" sounds awkward, it has become increasingly common in the celiac community.
3. Paul Starr, *The Social Transformation of American Medicine* (New York: Basic, 1982).
4. Nicholas A. Christakis, "The Ellipsis of Prognosis in Modern Medical Thought," *Social Science and Medicine* 44, no. 3 (1997): 301–15; Charles E. Rosenberg, "The Tyranny of Diagnosis: Specific Entities and Individual Experience," *Milbank Quarterly* 80, no. 2 (2002): 237–60.
5. Margot L. Herman et al., "Patients with Celiac Disease Are Not Followed Up Adequately," *Clinical Gastroenterology and Hepatology* 10 (2012): 893–99.
6. Eliot Freidson, *Professionalism, the Third Logic* (Chicago: University of Chicago Press, 2001), 127.
7. Nancy Tomes, *Remaking the American Patient: How Madison Avenue and Modern Medicine Turned Patients into Consumers* (Chapel Hill: University of North Carolina Press, 2016).
8. See, e.g., Marion Nestle, "Today's 'Eat More' Environment: The Rise of the Food Industry," in *A Place at the Table: The Crisis of 49 Million Hungry Americans and How to Solve It*, ed. Peter Pringle (New York: PublicAffairs, 2013), 95–106; Kelly D. Brownell, *Food Fight: The Inside Story of the Food Industry* (New York: McGraw Hill, 2004); David Kessler, *The End of Overeating: Taking Control of the Insatiable American Appetite* (Emmaus, PA: Rodale Press, 2009).
9. Anahad O'Connor, "New Dietary Guidelines Urge Less Sugar for All and Less Protein for Boys and Men," *New York Times*, January 7, 2016; see also James Jamblin, "How Agriculture Controls Nutrition Guidelines," *Atlantic*, October 6, 2015; Marion Nestle, *Food Politics: How the Food Industry Influences Nutrition and Health* (Berkeley: University of California Press, 2013). The guidelines affect the content of the school lunch program and the goals of national food-assistance programs.

10 Quoted in Philip F. Stahel, Todd F. VanderHeiden, and Fernanado J. Kim, "Why Do Surgeons Continue to Perform Unnecessary Surgery?," *Patient Safety in Surgery* 11, no. 1 (2017): 11.
11 Ishani Ganguli, "Cascades of Care after Incidental Findings in a U.S. National Survey of Physicians," *JAMA Network Open* 2, no. 10 (2019): e1913325.
12 Ryan Levi, "When Routine Medical Tests Trigger a Cascade of Costly, Unnecessary Care," *NPR*, July 14, 2022.
13 Heather Lyu, "Overtreatment in the United States," *PLoS One* 12, no. 9 (2017): e018970.
14 See Aaron E. Carroll, "The High Costs of Unnecessary Care," *Jamanetwork*, November 14, 2017.
15 Nestle, *Food Politics*, 2.
16 Alice Callahan, "Are We Close to a Treatment for Celiac Disease?," *New York Times*, June 1, 2022.
17 Sarah F. Rose, "Work," in *Keywords for Disability Studies*, ed. Rachel Adams, Benjamin Reiss, and David Serlin (New York: New York University Press, 2015), 187.
18 See Kathlyn Conway, *Beyond Words: Illness and the Limits of Expression* (Albuquerque: University of New Mexico Press, 2007).
19 Steven Lubet, "ME/CFS and Law Schools," *Faculty Lounge: Conversations about Law, Culture, and Academia*, November 2019, www.thefacultylounge.org.
20 Jessica Lebovits, "Impact of Celiac Disease on Dating," *Digestive Diseases and Sciences* 67, no. 11 (November 2022): 5158–67.
21 Paula Kamen, *All in My Head: An Epic Quest to Cure an Unrelenting, Totally Unreasonable, and Only Slightly Enlightening Headache* (Cambridge, MA: Da Capo, 2005), 70.
22 Cited in Jean E. Jackson, "Stigma, Liminality, and Chronic Pain: Mind-Body Borderlands," *American Ethnologist* 32 (August 2005): 341.
23 Lebovits, "Impact of Celiac Disease."
24 Eduardo Sabaté, *Adherence to Long-Term Therapies: Evidence for Action* (Geneva: World Health Organization, 2003), 3–4.
25 See, e.g., Gluten Dude, "What Happened to Celiac.com," *Gluten Dude*, November 1, 2019, https://glutendude.com.

CHAPTER 1. THE RISE AND FALL OF CELIAC DISEASE IN THE UNITED STATES

1 Samuel Gee, "On the Coeliac Affection," *St. Bartholomew's Report* 24 (1888): 17–21.
2 Sydney A. Halpern, *American Pediatrics: The Social Dynamics of Professionalism* (Berkeley: University of California Press, 1988), 36.
3 Halpern, *American Pediatrics*, 35–59.
4 Robert Luther Duffus and L. Emmett Holt Jr., *L. Emmett Holt, Pioneer of a Children's Century* (New York: D. Appleton-Century, 1940); Halpern, *American Pediatrics*, 62–65.

5   Emmett Holt, *The Diseases of Infancy and Childhood*, 6th ed. (New York: D. Appleton, 1914), 122.
6   See Rima D. Apple, *Perfect Motherhood: Science and Childrearing in America* (New Brunswick, NJ: Rutgers University Press, 2006), 35–38.
7   See Richard A. Meckel, *Save the Babies: American Public Health Reform and the Prevention of Infant Mortality, 1850–1929* (Baltimore, MD: Johns Hopkins University Press, 1990); Jacqueline H. Wolf, *Don't Kill Your Baby: Public Health and the Decline of Breastfeeding in the Nineteenth and Twentieth Centuries* (Columbus: Ohio State University Press, 2001).
8   The Babies' Hospital of the City of New York, *Annual Report* (New York: Babies' Hospital, 1989–1910).
9   Quoted in Wolf, *Don't Kill Your Baby*, 48.
10 See L. Emmett Holt, "Patient Records, 1901–1923," case numbers 4219, 4242, 5200, Archives and Special Collections, Columbia University Health Sciences Library, New York, NY.
11 See Meckel, *Save the Babies*, 40, 48–49, 93–94.
12 Jeffrey P. Brosco, "Weight Charts and Well Child Care: When the Pediatrician Became the Expert in Child Health," in *Formative Years: Children's Health in the United States, 1880–2000*, ed. Alexandra Minna Stern and Howard Markel (Ann Arbor: University of Michigan Press, 2002), 93–94.
13 A. Herter, *On Infantilism from Chronic Intestinal Infection Characterized by the Over-growth and Persistence of Flora of the Nursing Period: A Study of the Clinical Course, Bacteriology, Chemistry, and Therapeutics of Arrested Development in Infancy* (New York: Macmillan, 1908), 6, 8.
14 See Leonard G. Parsons, "Celiac Disease," *American Journal of Diseases of Children* 43 (1932): 1295–1346.
15 George Washington Corner, *A History of the Rockefeller Institute, 1901–1953: Origins and Growth* (New York: Rockefeller Institute Press, 1964), 98.
16 John Howland, "Prolonged Intolerance to Carbohydrates," *Transactions* 33 (1921): 11–19.
17 Howland, "Prolonged Intolerance."
18 Lee Forrest Hill, "Infant Feeding: Historical and Current," *Pediatric Clinic North America Journal* 14 (1967): 256.
19 Edwards A. Park, "John Howland Award Address," *Pediatrics* 2 (1953): 93.
20 Howland, "Prolonged Intolerance," 15.
21 Sidney V. Haas, "The Value of the Banana in the Treatment of Celiac Disease," *American Journal of Diseases of Children* 24 (1924): 421–37.
22 Emmett Holt, *The Care and Feeding of Children*, 2nd edition (New York: D. Appleton, 1897), 48–50.
23 Virginia Scott Jenkins, *Bananas: An American History* (Washington, DC: Smithsonian Institution Press, 2000); John Soluri, "Banana Cultures: Linking the Production and Consumption of Export Bananas, 1800–1980," in *Banana Wars:*

Power, Production, and History in the Americas, ed. Steve Striffler and Mark Moberg (Durham, NC: Duke University Press, 2003), 48–79.

24 Anon., *Food Value of the Banana: Opinion of Leading Medical and Scientific Authorities* (Boston: United Fruit Company, 1917).

25 Victor C. Myers and Anton R. Rose, "The Nutritional Value of the Banana," in Anon., *Food Value*, 17.

26 Anon., "Extract from *Journal of the American Medical Association*," in Anon., *Food Value*, 20.

27 Frank Crane, "Bananas One of the Chief Means of Sustenance to People of the Nation," in Anon., *Food Value*, 23.

28 Anon., "Opinion of Dr. Albert Harris How, Author of 'Eating and Drinking,'" in Anon., *Food Value*, 15.

29 Myers and Rose, "Nutritional Value," 15.

30 Anon., "Opinion of Dr. W. Gilman Thompson, Author of 'Practical Dietetics,'" in Anon., *Food Value*.

31 C. Pease and A. R. Rose, "Banana as a Food for Children," *American Journal of Diseases of Children* 14 (1917): 379.

32 Haas, "Value of the Banana," 421.

33 Haas, "Value of the Banana," 422.

34 Haas, "Value of the Banana," 423.

35 Harvey Levenstein, *Revolution at the Table: The Transformation of the American Diet* (Berkeley: University of California Press, 2003), 86–87.

36 Haas, "Value of the Banana," 421.

37 Haas, "Value of the Banana," 421.

38 Bertha M. Wood, "The Banana," *American Journal of Nursing* 28 (1928): 472.

39 Sidney V. Haas, "Powdered Ripe Banana in Infant Feeding," *Archives of Pediatrics* 48 (1931): 249.

40 Sidney V. Haas, "Celiac Disease: Its Specific Treatment and Cure without Nutritional Relapse," *Journal of the American Medical Association* 99 (1932): 448–52.

41 "New Vaccine Held Rheumatism in Check: Bananas Help Ill Child," *New York Times*, May 12, 1932.

42 John Lovett Morse, "Progress in Pediatrics," *New England Journal of Medicine* 204 (1932): 674.

43 Anon., *Food Value of the Banana*, 2nd edition (Boston: United Fruit Company, 1936).

44 Anon., *Nutritive and Therapeutic Value of the Banana: A Digest of Scientific Literature* (Boston: United Fruit Company, 1936).

45 Jenkins, *Bananas*, 95.

46 "24 Bananas for Baby, Ill of Rare Ailment, Are Located after Police Join Frantic Hunt," *New York Times*, July 31, 1942.

47 "Banana Priorities," *Newsweek*, August 10, 1942.

48 Sidney V. Haas, "Letter to the Editor," *New York Times*, August 4, 1942.
49 Ad at end of *American Journal of Nursing* 45 (1945).
50 Marcelo Bucheli and Ian Read, "Chronology," United Fruit Company, 2001, www.unitedfruit.org.
51 Ad at end of *American Journal of Nursing* 59 (1953).
52 *Golden Jubilee World Tribute to Dr. Sidney V. Haas in Honor of His Pioneering Contribution to Celiac Therapy and the Treatment of the Hypertonic Infant, and of the Completion of His Fiftieth Year of Medical Practice* (New York: Committee for the Golden Jubilee Tribute to Dr. Sidney V. Haas, 1949), 3.
53 Sidney V. Haas and Merrill P. Haas, "Diagnosis and Treatment of Celiac Disease," *Postgraduate Medicine* 7 (1950): 239–50.
54 P. van Berge-Henegouwen and C. J. Mulder, "Pioneer in the Gluten-Free Diet: William-Karel Dicke, 1905–1962," *Gut* 34, no. 11 (1993): 1473–75.
55 V. Haas, "Celiac Disease," *New York State Journal of Medicine* 63 (1963): 1347.
56 John Walker-Smith, "Historic Notes in Pediatric Gastroenterology: Margot Shiner, Coeliac Disease, and Small Intestinal Biopsy in Childhood," *Journal of Pediatric Gastroenterology & Nutrition* 25, no. 3 (September 1997): 316.
57 Emmett Holt Jr., Rustin McIntosh, and Henry L. Barnett, *Pediatrics*, 13th edition (New York: Appleton-Century-Crofts, 1962), 262.
58 John D. Lloyd-Still, "Where Have All the Celiacs Gone?," *Pediatrics* 61 (1978): 929–30.
59 Alessio Fasano, "Where Have All the American Celiacs Gone?," *Acta Pediatrica* 85 (May 1996): 20–24.
60 Searches were conducted through two article databases, Readers' Guide Retrospective and ProQuest.
61 Keith O'Brien, "Beat the Wheat," *New York Times*, November 27, 2011.
62 In 2013, when Fasano was appointed division chief of Pediatric Gastroenterology and Nutrition at Mass General Hospital for Children, he moved the Center for Celiac Research to Boston.
63 Fasano, "Where Have All the American Celiacs Gone?"
64 Alessio Fasano et al., "Prevalence of Celiac Disease in At-Risk and Not-at-Risk Groups in the United States," *Archives of Internal Medicine* 163 (2003): 286–92.
65 Quoted in Laura E. Derr, "When Food Is Poison: The History, Consequences, and Limitations of the Food Allergen Labeling and Consumer Protection Act of 2004," *Food and Drug Law Journal* 61, no. 1 (2006): 65–165, quotation on 102.
66 "National Institutes of Health Consensus Development Conference Statement on Celiac Disease, June 28–30, 2004," *Gastroenterology* 128 (2005): S1–S9.
67 Robert D. Zipser et al., "Brief Report: Physician Awareness of Celiac Disease: A Need for Further Education," *Journal of General Internal Medicine* 20, no. 7 (July 2005): 644–46.
68 "Celiac Centers, Labs & Alternative Resources," Beyond Celiac, www.beyondceliac.org, accessed February 13, 2024.

69 Andrew Perrin, "Social Media Usage: 2005–2015," Pew Research Center, October 8, 2015, www.pewresearch.org.

CHAPTER 2. GLUTEN-FREE FOOD

1 Euridice Martinez Steele et al., "Ultra-Processed Foods and Added Sugars in the U.S. Diet: Evidence from a Nationally Representative Cross-Sectional Study, *BMJ Open* 6 (2016); Mark Bittman, "Telling Americans to 'Eat Better' Doesn't Work: We Must Make Healthier Food," *Guardian*, December 4, 2022; Katherine D. McManus, "What Are Ultra-Processed Foods and Are They Bad for Our Health?," *Harvard Health*, January 2020.
2 Quoted in Michael Spector, "Against the Grain: Should You Go Gluten-Free?," *New Yorker*, November 3, 2014. See L. Fry, A. M. Madden, and R. Fallaize, "An Investigation into the Nutritional Composition and Cost of Gluten-Free versus Regular Food Products in the U.K.," *Journal of Human Nutrition and Dietetics* 31, no. 1 (2017): 108–20.
3 Keith O'Brien, "Should We All Go Gluten-Free?," *New York Times*, November 25, 2011.
4 NPD Group, "Percentage of U.S. Adults Trying to Cut Down or Avoid Gluten in Their Diets Reaches New High in 2013," NPD Press Release, March 6, 2013.
5 O'Brien, "Should We All Go Gluten Free?"
6 Cited in Jeffrey Kluger, "Eat More Gluten: The Diet Fad Must Die," *Time*, June 23, 2014.
7 Elaine Watson, "What's the Size of the US Gluten-Free Prize? $490m, $5bn, or $10bn?" *Food Navigator–USA*, February 17, 2014.
8 Quoted in Caroline Scott-Thomas, "Gluten-Free Trend Could Fall like 'a House of Cards,'" *Food Navigator–USA*, March 23, 2010.
9 Cited in Elaine Watson, "Culinary Tides: 'Not Only Have We Already Hit the Ceiling, the Gluten-Free Bubble Is Already Bursting,'" *Food Navigator–USA*, February 17, 2014.
10 Gill Hyslop, "Life after Gluten Free: What Will Happen to the Trend When Consumers Move on to 'The Next Best Thing'?," Bakery & Snacks, July 11, 2019, www.bakeryandsnacks.com.
11 Meticulous Research, "Gluten-Free Products Market to Reach $10.96 Billion by 2029: Exclusive Report by Meticulous Research," GlobeNewswire, April 6, 2022; Newsmantraa, "Non-Gluten Products Market Is Booming Worldwide, Nestle, General Mills, Raisio Group," *Digital Journal*, March 21, 2022; "Market Analysis Report: Gluten-Free Products Market Size, Share, and Trends Analysis," Grand View Research, March 2022.
12 Elaine Watson, "Health/Weight-Conscious Consumers Are Driving the Gluten-Free Market, Not Celiac," *FoodNavigator-USA*, October 14, 2013.
13 Warren J. Belasco, *Appetite for Change: How the Counterculture Took on the Food Industry* (Ithaca, NY: Cornell University Press, 2007), 175.

14 Quoted in Harvey Levenstein, *Paradox of Plenty: A Social History of Eating in Modern America* (Berkeley: University of California Press, 2003), 207–8.
15 Melinda Cooper, *Family Values: Between Neoliberalism and the New Social Conservatism* (New York: Zone Books, 2017), 101.
16 Watson, "Health/Weight Conscious Consumers."
17 Department of Health and Human Services, *The Surgeon General's Call to Action to Prevent and Decrease Overweight and Obesity, 2001* (Washington, DC: U.S. Government Printing Office), xiii–iv.
18 Charlotte Biltekoff, *Eating Right in America: The Cultural Politics of Food and Health* (Durham, NC: Duke University Press, 2013), 125.
19 Viren Swami, "Women's Idealized Bodies Have Changed Dramatically over Times—but Are Standards Becoming More Unattainable?," *Conversation*, September 13, 2016.
20 William Davis, *Wheat Belly: Lose the Wheat, Lose the Weight, and Find Your Path Back to Health*, revised and expanded edition (New York: Rodale, 2019), 3.
21 Davis, *Wheat Belly*, xii.
22 Davis, *Wheat Belly*, 12.
23 Davis, *Wheat Belly*, ix, 278.
24 Davis, *Wheat Belly*, 43, 103, 162.
25 David Perlmutter with Kristin Lorber, *Grain Brain: The Surprising Truth about Wheat, Carbs, and Sugar—Your Brain's Silent Killers* (New York: Little, Brown, Spark, 2018), quotations on 40 and 41.
26 Perlmutter, *Grain Brain*, quotations on 260 and 270.
27 See especially, Fred Brouns et al., "Do Ancient Wheats Contain Less Gluten Than Modern Bread Wheat, in Favour of Better Health?," *Nutrition Bulletin* 47, no. 2 (June 2022): 157–67; Donald D. Kasarda, "Can an Increase in Celiac Disease Be Attributed to an Increase in the Gluten Content of Wheat as a Consequence of Wheat Breeding?," *Journal of Agriculture and Food Chemistry* 61, no. 6 (2013): 1155–59.
28 "Wheat Belly Arguments Are Based on Shaky Science, Critics Say," *CBC News*, February 27, 2015; Julie Jones, "*Wheat Belly*: An Analysis of Selected Statements and Basic Theses from the Book," *Cereal Foods World* 57, no. 4 (July–August 2012): 177–87.
29 David T. Nash and Amy R. Slutzky," "Gluten Sensitivity: New Epidemic or New Myth? Every Major Change in Our Diet Carries with It the Possibility of Unforeseen Risks," *American Journal of Cardiology* 114 (2014): 1621–22.
30 Quoted in David Fryxell, "The Truth about the War on Wheat: Is This Dietary Staple Bad for Your Belly and Your Brain?," *Tufts Health and Nutrition Letter*, October 2, 2014; see Fred J. P. H. Brouns, Vincent J. van Buul, and Peter R. Shewry, "Does Wheat Make Us Fat and Sick?," *Journal of Cereal Science* 58 (2013): 209–15.
31 Davis, *Wheat Belly*, 83.

32 Perlmutter, *Grain Brain*, 60.
33 See Nicos Kefalas, "Self-Help and Self-Promotion: Dietary Advice and Agency in North America and Britain," in *Balancing the Self: Medicine, Politics, and the Regulation of Health in the Twentieth Century*, ed. Mark Jackson and Martin D. Moore (Manchester, UK: Manchester University Press, 2020).
34 Perlmutter, *Grain Brain*, 4.
35 Davis, *Wheat Belly*, x.
36 "A Slew of Cookbooks Have Been Published to Help Bakers Navigate a Gluten-Free Kitchen," *New York Times*, May 31, 2011.
37 Eryn Brown, "Miley Cyrus: 'Everyone Should Try No Gluten'; Experts Disagree," *Los Angeles Times*, April 10, 2012.
38 "Lady Gaga the Latest Celebrity to Go Gluten-Free," Beyond Celiac, August 23, 2012, www.beyondceliac.org.
39 Gretchen Reynolds, "When Athletes Go Gluten Free," *New York Times*, January 20, 2016.
40 David Shaftel, "Novak Djokovic: The Unloved Champion," *New York Times*, September 7, 2015; Akshay Sawai, "A Decade of Novak Djokovic, a Decade of Gluten Free Diet, and a Bizarre Test," *Money Control*, June 15, 2021, www.moneycontrol.com.
41 The Cartoon Bank, *New Yorker*, https://cartoonbank.com, accessed February 16, 2024.
42 Gluten Dude, "'Dear Elle,' about Your Awful Gluten-Free Cartoon," *Gluten Dude*, May 25, 2016, https://glutendude.com.
43 Gluten Dude, "Rachael Ray Calls Us Picky . . . Then Uses Gluten in a Gluten-Free Recipe," *Gluten Dude*, February 10, 2013, https://glutendude.com.
44 Carina Hoskisson, "Why Do Your Kid's Allergies Mean My Kid Can't Have a Birthday?," *HuffPost* Contributor platform, February 20, 2014.
45 Sophie Egan, "How Other People's Food Allergies Are Changing What You Eat," *Washington Post*, November 6, 2017.
46 Kristina Monllos, "Nearly 15,000 People Are Upset That Nascar's Super Bowl Ad Makes Fun of Being Gluten-Free," *Hollywood Reporter*, January 30, 2015; "CDF Comments on Gluten Danger Super Bowl Ad," Celiac Disease Foundation, January 31, 2015, https://celiac.org.
47 "Barstool Sports: 'Gluten-Free People Are Weak and Pathetic,'" Gluten Dude, February 8, 2022, https://glutendude.com.
48 Michelle Castillo, "Disney Pulls 'Jessie' Episode That Makes Fun of Gluten-Free Child," *CBS News*, May 20, 2013.
49 Katie Reilly, "Ted Cruz Pledges Not to Provide Gluten-Free Meals to the Military," *Time*, February 16, 2016.
50 Video available on Jon Bari, "Hoda Kotb and Joy Behar, 'Why You Gotta Be So Mean?,'" Celiac Journey, May 12, 2022, www.celiacjourney.com.
51 Quoted in Salamishah Tillet, "Filmmakers with a Focus on Justice," *New York Times*, July 1, 2020.

52 Tim Arango, "Old Riots, New Pain: Recalling the Past in Los Angeles," *New York Times*, June 4, 2020.
53 Jenny Kutner, "'SNL' Brilliantly Tackles Gentrification: 'You're Acting Like Someone Put Gluten in Your Muffin,'" *Salon*, January 18, 2015.
54 "Jimmy Kimmel Asks: Just What Is Gluten Anyway?," *Los Angeles Times*, May 8, 2014.
55 Monika Laszkowska et al., "Socioeconomic vs. Health-Related Factors Associated with Good Searches for Gluten-Free Diet," *Clinical Gastroenterology and Hepatology* 16 (2018): 295–97.
56 Harvey Levenstein, *Fear of Food: A History of Why We Worry about What We Eat* (Chicago: University of Chicago Press, 2012), 4.
57 Quoted in Ellen McCarthy, "Backlash Has Begun against Gluten-Free Dieters," *Washington Post*, July 6, 2014.
58 Kluger, "Eat More Gluten."
59 McCarthy, "Backlash."
60 Neil Swidey, "Why Food Allergy Fakers Need to Stop: From Gluten to Garlic, Diets and Dislikes Are Being Passed Off as Medical Conditions; Chefs and Real Sufferers Have Had Enough," *Boston Globe*, October 14, 2015.
61 April Peveteaux, "Tavern on the Green Already Sucked," Gluten Is My Bitch, May 1, 2011, https://glutenismybitch.com.
62 Swidey, "Food Allergy Fakers."
63 Priyanka Chugh, "Open Letter to Jimmy Fallon," Opnlttr, September 5, 2015, https://opnlttr.com. The video is available on "Jimmy Fallon . . . What Did We Ever Do to You?," *Gluten Dude*, November 20, 2013, https://glutendude.com.
64 Quoted in Gluten Dude, "Disney Thinks Bullying a Gluten Free Child Is Funny," *Gluten Dude*, May 16, 2013, https://glutendude.com.
65 Castillo, "Disney Pulls 'Jessie' Episode."
66 Monllos, "Nearly 15,000 People Are Upset."
67 "The Today Show Apologizes to the Gluten-Free Community . . . Sort Of," *Gluten Dude*, May 29, 2013, https://glutendude.com.
68 "'Dear Elle.'"
69 See Amy Trubek, *Making Modern Meals: How Americans Cook Today* (Berkeley: University of California Press, 2017), 195.
70 Rachael Rettner, "Most People Shouldn't Eat Gluten-Free," *Scientific American*, March 11, 2013; Emily B. Rubin, Melissa R. Viscuso, and Stephanie M. Moleski, "Maintaining a Balanced Diet while Gluten-Free: Treatment Options," *Current Treatment Options in Gastroenterology* 18 (2020): 699–717; Charlene Elliott, "The Nutritional Quality of Gluten-Free Products for Children," *Pediatrics* 142, no. 2 (2018): 1–8; James Hamblin, "The Harm in Blindly 'Going Gluten Free': It Is Not an Innocuous Decision," *Atlantic*, May 2016; Timmaiah G. Theethira and Melinda Dennis, "Celiac Disease and the Gluten-Free Diet: Consequences and Recommendations for Improvement," *Digestive Diseases* 33 (2015): 175–82; Giorgia

Vici, Luca Belli, Massimiliano Biondi, and Valerie Polzonnetti, "Gluten Free Diet and Nutrient Deficiencies: A Review," *Clinical Nutrition* 35, no. 6 (2016); Valentina Melini and Francesca Melini, "Gluten-Free Diet: Gaps and Needs for a Healthier Diet," *Nutrients* 11, no. 1 (January 2019): 170.

71 See Stephanie L. Raehsler et al., "Accumulation of Heavy Metals in People on a Gluten-Free Diet," *Clinical Gastroenterology and Hepatology* 16 (2018): 244–51; Nicholas Bakalar, "A Downside of Gluten Free," *New York Times*, February 16, 2017.

72 Neil Swidey, "How We Made Gluten into a Monster: A Pioneering Celiac Doctor Explains the Misguided Origins of 'the Most popular Diet That You Can Imagine,'" *Boston Globe*, October 27, 2015.

73 Cited in "Wheat Belly Arguments."

74 See Abigail M. Okrent and Aylin Kumcu, "U.S. Households' Demand for Convenience Foods," U.S. Department of Agriculture Research Service, July 2016, www.ers.usda.gov.

75 "A Gluten-Free Diet: How Much Will It Cost You?" *CBS News*, February 25, 2014, www.cbsnews.com.

76 Y. Zhang Verrill and R. Kane, "Food Label Usage and Reported Difficulty with Following a Gluten-Free Diet among Individuals in the USA with Coeliac Disease and Those with Noncoeliac Gluten Sensitivity," *Journal of Human Nutrition and Dietetics* 26 (2013): 479–87.

77 Jennifer Esposito, *Jennifer's Way* (Boston: Da Capo, 2014), 154.

78 Melissa Clark, "Gluten-Free Flavor-Free No More," *New York Times*, May 31, 2011.

79 Keith O'Brien, "Beat the Wheat: How Getting the Gluten out of Chex Cereals Helped Turn a Marketing Niche into a Mainstream Phenomenon," *New York Times*, November 27, 2011.

80 Anne R. Lee, Randi L. Wolf, Benjamin Lebwohl, Edward J. Ciaccio, and Peter H. R. Green, "Persistent Economic Burden of the Gluten Free Diet," *Nutrients* 11, no. 2 (February 14, 2019).

81 Lee, Wolf, Lebwohl, Ciaccio, and Green, "Persistent Economic Burden."

82 Marion Nestle, *Food Politics: How the Food Industry Influences Nutrition and Health*, revised and expanded edition (Berkeley: University of California Press, 2013), 17.

83 Michael Moss, *Salt, Sugar, and Fat* (New York: Random House, 2014), 341. See also Ashley Gearhardt et al., "Social, Clinical, and Policy Implications of Ultra-processed Food Addiction," *BMJ* 2023: 383:e075354.

84 World Health Organization, Executive Summary, in *Food Marketing Exposure and Power and Their Association with Food-Related Attitudes, Beliefs, and Behaviours: A Narrative Review* (World Health Organization, 2022).

85 Quoted in Stephanie Strom, "A Big Bet on Gluten-Free," *New York Times*, February 17, 2014.

86 Trubek, *Making Modern Meals*, 67–68.

87 Elizabeth Sloan, "What, When, and Where America Eats," *Food Technology Magazine*, January 1, 2020, www.ift.org.
88 Laura Shapiro, *Something from the Oven: Reinventing Dinner in 1950s America* (New York: Penguin, 2004), pp. xxi–xxii.
89 Juliet B. Schor, *The Overworked American: The Unexpected Decline of Leisure* (New York: Basic Books, 1992). But see Judy Wajcman, *Pressed for Time: The Acceleration of Life in Digital Capitalism* (Chicago: University of Chicago Press, 2015), 63–64.
90 Alexander Bick, Bettina Brüggemann, and Nicola Fuchs-Schündeln, "Hours Worked in Europe and the U.S.: New Data, New Answers," CEPR Discussion Paper No. DP11483, SSRN, August 2016, https://ssm.com; Jody Heymann and Alison Earle, *Raising the Global Floor: Dismantling the Myth That We Can't Afford Good Working Conditions for Everyone* (Stanford, CA: Stanford University Press, 2010).
91 Arlie Hochschild with Anne Machung, *The Second Shift: Working Parents and the Revolution at Home* (New York: Viking, 1989); Suzanne M. Bianchi, Melissa A. Milkie, Liana C. Sayer, and John P. Robinson, "Is Anyone Doing the Housework? Trends in the Gender Division of Household Labor," *Social Forces* 79 (September 2000): 191–228; see Maureen Perry-Jenkins and Naomi Gerstel, "Work and Family in the Second Decade of the 21st Century," *Journal of Marriage and the Family* 82 (February 2020): 420–53.

CHAPTER 3. IS IT REALLY GLUTEN FREE?

1 MSTEM, "Media Diet Lessons from the Embattled History of Nutrition Labels," Civic Media, MIT, https://civic.mit.edu; see Institute of Medicine, *Front-of-Package Nutrition Rating Systems and Symbols: Promoting Healthier Choices* (Washington, DC: National Academies Press, 2012), chapter 4.
2 See Steve L. Taylor, "Emerging Problems with Food Allergies," Food and Agriculture Organization of the United Nations, 2000, www.fao.org.
3 Matthew Smith, *Another Person's Poison: A History of Food Allergy* (New York: Columbia University Press, 2015), 152–85.
4 William R. Greer "Consumer Saturday: Warnings on Food Allergies," *New York Times*, March 29, 1986.
5 In 2012 FAAN merged with the Food Allergy Initiative (FAI) to become Food Allergy Research and Education (FARE).
6 Kelly Thomas, "School Lunches for Allergy-Prone Youth Take Planning," *Orange County Register*, September 13, 2000.
7 Smith, *Another Person's Poison*.
8 Constance L. Hays, "Allergic Reactions to Nuts Are Dangerous to Millions," *New York Times*, February 22, 1998.
9 Laura E. Derr, "When Food Is Poison: The History, Consequences, and Limitations of the Food Allergen Labeling and Consumer Protection Act of 2004," *Food and Drug Law Journal* 61, no. 1 (2006): 80.

10 Quoted in Derr, "When Food Is Poison," 81.
11 "FDA Survey Finds Faulty Listing of Possible Food Allergies," *New York Times*, April 3, 2001.
12 Derr, "When Food Is Poison," 81–87.
13 Derr, "When Food Is Poison," 110.
14 Alison Kretser, "Food Allergen Labels," Letter to Editor, *New York Times*, June 2, 2003.
15 Philip Brasher, "Allergy-Inducing Foods Will Soon Get New Labeling," *Philadelphia Tribune*, June 8, 2001.
16 "Industry Sets Guidelines for Clearer Food Labels," *Washington Post*, May 31, 2001.
17 Greg Winter, "Calls for Increasing Clarity on Food Labels," *New York Times*, July 2, 2002.
18 Quoted in Winter, "Calls for Increasing Clarity."
19 Quoted in Derr, "When Food Is Poison," 107; see "Food Industry Opposing Label Improvements," Center for Science in the Public Interest, September 20, 2002, www.cspinet.org.
20 Jax Peters Lowell, *The Gluten-Free Bible* (New York: St. Martin's Griffin, 2005), 440.
21 Quoted in Derr, "When Food Is Poison," 102.
22 Quoted in Jon Bari, "Gluten Should Be Labeled as a Top Food Allergen in the U.S., Just Like in Canada and across Europe," Celiac Journey, July 7, 2021, 5, www.celiacjourney.com.
23 Quoted in Bari, "Gluten Should Be Labeled," 11.
24 Quoted in Bari, "Gluten Should Be Labeled," 11.
25 "Substitute Pulls Mandatory Gluten Declaration: Senate Panel Passes Watered-Down Food Allergen Labeling Bill," *Inside Washington's FDA Week* 8, no. 39 (September 27, 2002): 5.
26 Quoted in Derr, "When Food Is Poison," 145.
27 Quoted in Derr, "When Food Is Poison," 143.
28 Quoted in Derr, "When Food Is Poison," 142.
29 Derr, "When Food Is Poison," 152.
30 D. T. Thompson, A. Keller, and T. B. Lyons, "When Foods Contain Both a Gluten-free Claim and an Allergen Advisory Statement for Wheat: Should Consumers Be Concerned?," *European Journal of Clinical Nutrition* 72 (2018): 931–35.
31 "Three Years Later, What Is the Impact of the Gluten-Free Labeling Standard? A Conversation with Carol D'Lima and Alessio Fasano," U.S. Food and Drug Administration, October 4, 2017, www.fda.gov.
32 Department of Health and Human Services, Food and Drug Administration, 21 CFR Part 101, Docket no. FDA-2005-N-0404, *Federal Register* 78, no. 150 (August 5, 2013): 47157.

33 Quoted in "Gluten Free Standards Draw Criticism by Consumer Group, Industry," *Inside Washington's FDA Week* 13, no. 4 (January 26, 2007): 12.
34 Quoted in "Gluten Food Standards Draw Criticism," 12.
35 Quoted in "Gluten Free Standards Draw Criticism," 12.
36 See Caroline Scott-Thomas, "FDA Reopens Comments on Gluten-Free Labeling," *Food Navigator–USA*, August 2, 2011, www.foodnavigator-usa.com.
37 Quoted in Jane E. Allen, "Activists Protest Delayed Gluten-Free Label Standard," ABC New Medical Unit, May 3, 2011, https://abcnews.go.com.
38 Quoted in Lyndsey Layton, "3 Years after Deadline, FDA Still Hasn't Defined 'Gluten-Free,'" *Washington Post*, April 28, 2011.
39 Dyani Barber, "Paul Seelig Found Guilty of Selling Fake Gluten-Free Bread Gets 11 Years," Celiac.com, April 12, 2011, www.celiac.com; Layton, "3 Years"; "Durham Bread Company Owner Sentenced for Fraud," *WRAL News*, April 12, 2011, www.wral.com.
40 Allen, "Activists Protest."
41 Layton, "3 Years."
42 Quoted in Allen, "Activists Protest."
43 Marion Nestle, *Food Politics: How the Food Industry Influences Nutrition and Health* (Berkeley: University of California Press, 2013), 101–2; Elizabeth Flock, "Monsanto Petition Tells Obama: 'Cease FDA Ties to Monsanto,'" *Washington Post*, January 30, 2012; "Tell Obama to Cease FDA Ties to Monsanto," campaign created by Frederick Ravid, https://sign.moveon.org; Rebecca Trager, "Obama Urged to Cut FDA Ties with Monsanto," Cornucopia Institute, February 9, 2012.
44 Nestle, *Food Politics*, 101.
45 Flock, "Monsanto Petition."
46 "Wyden, Leahy Letter Asks FDA for Gluten-Free Food Standards," Press Release, Ron Wyden: United States Senator for Oregon, July 21, 2011, www.wyden.senate.gov.
47 Quoted in Scott-Thomas, "FDA Reopens Comments."
48 Editorial Board, "Is It Really Gluten Free?," *New York Times*, August 15, 2013.
49 "4 Takeaways from Our Investigation into the FDA's Byzantine Food Arm," *Politico*, April 9, 2022.
50 "4 Takeaways."
51 DHHS, *Federal Register* (August 5, 2013), 47157.
52 Nestle, *Food Politics*, 95–110.
53 Quoted in Sabrina Tavernise, "FDA Sets a Standard on Labeling 'Gluten Free,'" *New York Times*, August 2, 2013.
54 See "Gluten-Free Labeling Compliance," Celiac Disease Foundation, October 31, 2014, https://celiac.org.
55 Tricia Thompson, "Action Alert: Notifying the FDA about Misbranded Gluten-Free Products," Gluten Free Watchdog, July 8, 2014, www.glutenfreewatchdog.org.
56 Tricia Thompson, "Help Stop Labeling Violations under the Gluten-Free Rule," Gluten Free Watchdog, August 23, 2017, www.glutenfreewatchdog.org.

57 Tricia Thompson, "Spot a Labeled Gluten-Free Food That's Misbranded? Here's What to Do," Gluten Free Watchdog, February 20, 2018, www.glutenfreewatchdog.org.
58 Tricia Thompson, "Enough Is Enough with Gluten-Free Misbranding: Contact FDA Today," Gluten Free Watchdog, February 17, 2020, www.glutenfreewatchdog.org.
59 Tricia Thompson, "Dietitians: Please Join Dietitians in Gluten and Gastrointestinal Disorders and Send a Letter to FDA Voicing Your Displeasure about the Lack of Enforcement of the Gluten-Free Labeling Rule," Gluten Free Watchdog, February 23, 2020, www.glutenfreewatchdog.org.
60 Tricia Thompson, "Four of Eight Products Recalled: YOU Are Making a Difference!," Gluten Free Watchdog, March 20, 2020, www.glutenfreewatchdog.org.
61 Tricia Thompson, "Plea to FDA: Turn Your Attention to the Manufacturers Who Blatantly Use Fermented and Hydrolyzed Wheat or Barley Ingredients in Labeled Gluten-Free Foods," Gluten Free Watchdog, July 13, 2020, www.glutenfreewatchdog.org.
62 Tricia Thompson, "Chef Myron's Sauces Containing Wheat-Based Soy Sauce FINALLY Recalled," Gluten Free Watchdog, January 4, 2021, www.glutenfreewatchdog.org.
63 Tricia Thompson, "Dandy Blend Instant Herbal Beverage: Where Is the Enforcement, FDA?," Gluten Free Watchdog, February 17, 2021, www.glutenfreewatchdog.org.
64 Tricia Thompson, "Does FDA Ever Intend to Take Public Enforcement Action against Manufacturers Misbranding Products Gluten-Free That List Malt Ingredients?," Gluten Free Watchdog, May 24, 2022, www.glutenfreewatchdog.org.
65 Comments submitted to FDA by Tricia Thompson, Adam Rapp, and Kaki Schmidt in response to public docket No. FDA-2023-N-2393, www.glutenfreewatchdog.org, accessed February 15, 2024.
66 Paul Starr, *The Social Transformation of American Medicine* (New York: Basic, 1982).

CHAPTER 4. PATIENT ADVOCACY, CORPORATE FUNDING, AND THE CHEERIOS DEBACLE

1 Matthew S. McCoy et al., "Conflicts of Interest for Patient-Advocacy Organizations," *New England Journal of Medicine* 376 (March 2, 2017): 880–85. The study also found that 39 percent of the organizations had a current or former industry executive on their board.
2 Gardiner Harris, "Drug Makers Are Advocacy Group's Biggest Donors," *New York Times*, October 21, 2009.
3 McCoy et al., "Conflicts of Interest."
4 Sheila M. Rothman, Victoria H. Ravels, Anne Friedman, and David J. Rothman, "Health Advocacy Organizations and the Pharmaceutical Industry: An Analysis of Disclosure Practices," *American Journal of Public Health* 101 (April 2011): 602.

5 Orla O'Donovan, "Corporate Colonization of Health Activism? Irish Health Advocacy Organizations' Modes of Engagement with Pharmaceutical Corporations," *International Journal of Health Services* 37, no. 4 (2007): 711–33.
6 McCoy et al., "Conflicts of Interest."
7 Philip Brasher, "Allergy-Inducing Foods Will Soon Get New Labeling," *Philadelphia Tribune*, June 8, 2001; "Food Allergies Stir a Mother to Action," *New York Times*, January 9, 2008.
8 Marc Santora, "In Diabetes Fight, Raising Cash and Keeping Trust," *New York Times*, November 25, 2008.
9 "Certified Gluten-Free," Gluten Intolerance Group, https://gluten.org, accessed February 15, 2024.
10 *Annual Report 2022*, 7, Gluten Intolerance Group, https://gluten.org, accessed February 18, 2024.
11 National Celiac Association Inc., Nonprofit Explorer—ProPublica, https://projects.propublica.org, accessed February 15, 2024.
12 *2022 Annual Report*, Celiac Disease Foundation, https://celiac.org, accessed February 15, 2024.
13 "About Beyond Celiac," Beyond Celiac, www.beyondceliac.org, accessed February 15, 2024.
14 *Annual Report for 2022*, 17, Beyond Celiac, www.beyondceliac.org, accessed February 16, 2024.
15 "About the Gluten Free Dietitian, Tricia Thompson," Gluten Free Dietician, www.glutenfreedietitian.com, accessed February 16, 2024.
16 "9 Meters Discontinues Phase 3 Trial for Potential Celiac Disease Drug Larazotide," Celiac Disease Foundation, June 21, 2022, https://celiac.org.
17 Verónica Segura et al., "New Insights into Non-Dietary Treatment in Celiac Disease: Emerging Therapeutic Options," *Nutrients* 13 (2021): 21–46; Tessa Dickman, Frits Koning, and Gerd Bouma, "Celiac Disease: New Therapies on the Horizon," *Current Opinion in Pharmacology* 66 (2022); Alice Callahan, "Are We Close to a Treatment for Celiac Disease?," *New York Times*, June 1, 2022.
18 Shah Sveta et al., "Patient Perception of Treatment Burden Is High in Celiac Disease Compared to Other Common Conditions," *American Journal of Gastroenterology* 109, no. 9 (September 2014): 1304–11.
19 Dennis De Leon Morilla et al., "Patients' Risks Tolerance for Non-Dietary Therapies in Celiac Disease," *Clinical Gastroenterology and Hepatology* 20 (2022): 2647–49.
20 Steven Epstein, "Measuring Success: Scientific, Institutional, and Cultural Effects of Patient Advocacy," in *Patients as Policy Actors*, ed. Beatrix Hoffman, Nancy Tomes, Rachel Grob, and Mark Schlesinger (New Brunswick, NJ: Rutgers University Press, 2011), 261.
21 "Impact of My PCORI Panel Appointment: Marilyn's Message, October 2021," Celiac Disease Foundation, November 22, 2021, https://celiac.org.

22 "Patient Recruitment Services," Celiac Disease Foundation, https://celiac.org, accessed June 8, 2023.
23 Celiac Disease Foundation, email message to author, April 27, 2023.
24 "Our Science Plan, Barriers to a Cure for Celiac Disease," Beyond Celiac, www.beyondceliac.org, accessed February 16, 2024.
25 Callahan, "Are We Close."
26 Celiac Disease Foundation, email message to author, April 27, 2023.
27 Michael Bérubé, *Life as Jamie Knows It: An Exceptional Child Grows Up* (Boston: Beacon, 2016), 83.
28 Emily Kopp, Sydney Lupkin, and Elizabeth Lucas, "Patient Advocacy Groups Take in Millions from Drugmakers: Is There a Payback?" *Kaiser Health News*, April 6, 2016.
29 "When Sponsorship Dollars Muddy the Messaging for Products Sold to the Gluten-Free Community," Gluten Free Watchdog, May 29, 2017, www.glutenfreewatchdog.org.
30 Indeed, Beyond Celiac's website asserts that in addition to fostering research, the organization focuses on "promoting the growth of the gluten-free industry" ("Sponsorship & Advertising Opportunities with Beyond Celiac," Beyond Celiac, www.beyondceliac.org, accessed February 16, 2024). The website also features numerous recipes provided by food-industry sponsors and incorporating their products ("Gluten Free Recipes," Beyond Celiac, www.beyondceliac.org, accessed March 10, 2023).
31 Jax Peters Lowell, *The Gluten-Free Bible* (New York: St. Martin's Griffin, 2005), 440.
32 Tricia Thompson, "Gluten-Free Community, This Is Your Chance! Let's Make Some Noise! Contact Your Members of Congress Today," Gluten Free Watchdog, August 2021, www.glutenfreewatchdog.org.
33 *2023 Annual Report*, Celiac Disease Foundation, December 2023, https://celiac.org.
34 "Proud Sponsors and Research Partners," Celiac Disease Foundation, https://celiac.org, accessed February 16, 2024.
35 "Gluten-Free Foods," Celiac Disease Foundation, https://celiac.org, accessed February 16, 2023.
36 Jennifer W. Cadenhead et al., "Diet Quality, Ultra-processed Food Consumption, and Quality of Life in a Cross-Sectional Cohort of Adults and Teens with Celiac Disease," *Journal of Human Nutrition and Dietetics* 36, no. 4 (August 2023): 1144–58, https://doi.org/10.1111/jhn.13137.
37 "Eat! Gluten Free on the App Store," Apple App Store, https://apps.apple.com, accessed February 24, 2024.
38 "Jessica's Natural Food," Celiac Disease Foundation, https://celiac.org, accessed February 16, 2024.

39 "Breakfast Sausage Egg Muffins," Celiac Disease Foundation, https://celiac.org, accessed February 16, 2024.
40 Cited in Marcia DeLonge and Karen Perry Stillman, *Champions of Breakfast: How Cereal-Makers Can Help Save Our Soil, Support Farmers, and Take a Bite out of Climate Change* (Cambridge, MA.: Union of Concerned Scientists, 2019), 4. The other major companies are the Kellogg Company, Post Consumer Brands, and Quaker Oats, a division of PepsiCo.
41 Cited in Marion Nestle, "Regulating the Food Industry: An Aspirational Agenda," *American Journal of Public Health* 112, no. 6 (June 2022): 853–58.
42 "Overview of the IOM Report on 'Food Marketing to Children and Youth: Threat or Opportunity?,'" Fact Sheet, Institute of Medicine, December 2005, https://nepc.colorado.edu.
43 "Cereal FACTS: Evaluating the Nutrition Quality and Marketing of Children's Cereals," Yale Rudd Center for Food Policy and Obesity, October 1, 2009, www.cerealfacts.org.
44 Jennifer Harris et al., "Cereal FACTS 2012: Limited Progress in the Nutrition Quality and Marketing of Children's Cereals," Yale Rudd Center for Food Policy and Obesity, June 2012, www.cerealfacts.org.
45 Warren J. Belasco, *Appetite for Change: How the Counterculture Took on the Food Industry* (Ithaca, NY: Cornell University Press, 1989).
46 Abigail Carroll, *Three Squares: The Invention of the American Meal* (New York: Basic Books, 2013).
47 David Leonard, "Who Killed Tony the Tiger?" *Businessweek*, February 26, 2015.
48 NPD research cited in Vanessa Wong, "Can an Old-School Cereal Giant Ride the Gluten-Free Wave?," *Buzzfeed*, September 13, 2015.
49 See Laura E. Derr, "When Food Is Poison: The History, Consequences, and Limitations of the Food Allergen Labeling and Consumer Protection Act of 2004," *Food and Drug Law Journal* 61, no. 1 (2006): 89; Matthew Smith, *Another Person's Poison: A History of Food Allergy* (New York: Columbia University Press, 2013), 171; Marilyn Chase, "Food-Product Labels Do a Sketchy Job of Helping the Allergic," *Wall Street Journal*, July 12, 1999; Susan Dominus, "The Allergy Prison," *New York Times*, June 10, 2001.
50 Quoted in Wong, "Can an Old-School Cereal Giant"; see Patricia A. Curtin, "General Mills: [Re]manufacturing the Gluten-Free Consumer Community," in *Public Relations and Participatory Culture: Fandom, Social Media, and Community Engagement*, ed. Amber L. Hutchins and Natalie T. J. Tindall (New York: Routledge, 2016), 119–31.
51 O'Brien, "Should We All Go Gluten-Free?"
52 Curtin, "General Mills."
53 Barbara Murray, "General Mills to Buy Small Planet Foods," *Supermarket News*, January 3, 2000, www.supermarketnews.com.

54 Elaine Watson, "General Mills Boosts Natural Foods Portfolio with Gluten Free Snacks Deal," *Food Navigator*, March 1, 2012.
55 "Marketing Mix of Cheerios," Marketing91, www.marketing91.com, accessed February 16, 2024.
56 Wong, "Can an Old School Cereal Giant."
57 See "More Thoughts on Gluten-Free Cheerios," Gluten Free Watchdog, May 6, 2015, www.glutenfreewatchdog.org.
58 Marion Nestle, "Lower Your Cholesterol with Cheerios? Oh Please," *Food Politics* blog, September 15, 2007.
59 Sally Greenberg, "Crack Down on Mislabeled Cheerios Welcome Action by FDA," National Consumers League, May 13, 2009, https://nclnet.org.
60 "General Mills Faces Suit for Making Bogus Claims about Cheerios," Westlaw, July 16, 2009, https://content.next.westlaw.com.
61 Marion Nestle, "Winter Friday: A Good Day for GMO Announcements," *Food Politics* blog, January 3, 2014, www.foodpolitics.com. Another incident occurred after gluten-free Cheerios began to reach supermarkets. In November 2015, CSPI and two law firms filed a lawsuit seeking to stop GM's "false and misleading marketing practices with regard to Cheerios Protein." The plaintiffs charged that the new cereal contained only slightly more protein than the original Cheerios but had seventeen times as much sugar per serving, which GM did not disclose. The settlement agreement reached in July 2018 required GM to stop exaggerating the protein content on the front of Cheerios Protein boxes and to state more clearly that the cereal was sweetened ("General Mills: Cheerios Protein," Center for Science in the Public Interest, updated October 8, 2021, www.cspinet.org).
62 "Stop Eating Gluten Free Foods," Gluten Dude, October 18, 2012, https://glutendude.com.
63 "Will the New Cheerios Really Be Gluten-Free? I'm About to Find Out," Gluten Dude, March 18, 2015, https://glutendude.com.
64 "The (Gluten-Free) Scoop on Cheerios," Beyond Celiac, March 26, 2015, www.beyondceliac.org.
65 "Marilyn's Message October 2015," Celiac Disease Foundation, October 13, 2015, https://celiac.org.
66 Gluten Dude, "Gluten-Free Cheerios? Here's the Deal," *Gluten Dude*, March 31, 2015, https://glutendude.com.
67 Tricia Thompson, "Gluten-Free Oat Production: Purity Protocol versus Mechanical or Optical Sorting; Does It Matter to You?," Gluten Free Watchdog, June 17, 2015, www.glutenfreewatchdog.org.
68 Comments, "Gluten-Free Cheerios: Take Two," Gluten Free Watchdog, updated July 22, 2015, www.glutenfreewatchdog.org.
69 Debi Smith, "Pissing in the Gluten-Free Cheerios," *Hunters Lyonesse* blog, August 20, 2015, https://hunterslyonesse.wordpress.com.

70 "Dear General Mills, about Your 'Gluten-Free' Cheerios," *In Johanna's Kitchen* blog, September 29, 2015, https://injohnnaskitchen.com.
71 Comments, "Gluten Free Cheerios: Take Two," Gluten Free Watchdog, updated August 14, 2015, www.glutenfreewatchdog.org.
72 Comments, "Gluten Free Cheerios: Take Two," updated August 14, 2015.
73 Quoted in Gluten Dude, "The Cheerios Recall (aka . . . The Gluten-Free Sh*t Storm)," *Gluten Dude*, October 2, 2015, https://glutendude.com.
74 Alice Bast, "Cheerios Recall: The Celiac Disease Community Is Constantly At-Risk," *Huffpost Life*, October 8, 2015.
75 Erin Smith, "Cheerios Update: Phone Call with General Mills," *Gluten-Free Fun* blog, September 16, 2015.
76 Phil Wahba, "General Mills Places Big Bet on Gluten-Free Cheerios," *Fortune*, September 22, 2015.
77 Anjali Athavaley and Ramkumar Iyer, "General Mills Is Recalling 1.8 Million Boxes of Gluten-Free Cheerios," *Business Insider*, October 5, 2015.
78 Elahe Izadi, "General Mills Recalls 1.8M Boxes of Gluten-Free Cheerios That May Not Be Gluten Free," *Washington Post*, October 6, 2015.
79 Izadi, "General Mills Recalls."
80 Erin Smith, "Cheerios Recall and 10 Reasons I Am Mad at General Mills," *Gluten-Free Fun* blog, October 6, 2015, https://glutenfreefun.blogspot.com.
81 Shirley Braden, "Stop Eating 'Gluten-Free' Cheerios Plus 9 More Thoughts on This Appalling Situation," *Gluten Free Easily*, October 6, 2015, https://glutenfreeeasily.com.
82 "Cheerios Are Not Gluten-Free," Alive Without Gluten, October 2015, www.alivewithoutgluten.com.
83 Tricia Thompson, "Open Letter to General Mills' Gluten-Free Cheerios Team on Behalf of the Gluten Free Watchdog Community," Gluten Free Watchdog, October 7, 2015, www.glutenfreewatchdog.org.
84 Quoted in Izadi, "General Mills Recalls."
85 "Marilyn's Message October 2015"; "General Mills Issues Voluntary Class 1 Recall of Cheerios and Honey Nut Cheerios Cereal Produced at Its Lodi, California Location on Certain Dates," Celiac Disease Foundation, October 5, 2015, https://celiac.org; "FDA Investigates Complaints Associated with Cheerios Labeled Gluten Free: General Mills Voluntarily Recalls Affected Lots," Celiac Disease Foundation, October 7, 2015, https://celiac.org.
86 Quoted in Vanessa Wong, "Cheerios Sales Are Growing after Switch to Gluten Free," *Buzzfeed News*, December 21, 2015.
87 Vanessa Wong, "'Not Safe for Celiacs': Gluten Free Cheerios Are Still Drawing Complaints," *Buzzfeed News*, July 6, 2017.
88 "Cheerios Recall Facts," gf Jules, https://gfjules.com, accessed April 9, 2023.
89 Quoted in Wong, "'Not Safe for Celiacs.'"

90 Quoted in Gluten Dude, "Gluten-Free Cheerios? NOT Recommended by the CCA," *Gluten Dude,* August 9, 2016, https://glutendude.com.
91 Wong, "'Not Safe for Celiacs.'"
92 Gluten Dude, "Should Celiac 'Leaders' Be Promoting Gluten Free(ish) Cheerios?," *Gluten Dude,* June 20, 2017, https://glutendude.com.
93 Quoted in "Should Celiac 'Leaders.'"
94 "Should Celiac 'Leaders.'"
95 Quoted in "Should Celiac 'Leaders.'"
96 See "Gluten Free vs. Gluten Friendly," Fat Celiac, September 18, 2020, https://fatceliac.net.
97 Quoted in Gluten Dude, "Gluten-FRIENDLY Brownie Mix? Gluten-FRIENDLY Biscuits? No GM. Just No," *Gluten Dude,* February 5, 2020, https://glutendude.com.
98 Quoted in "Gluten-FRIENDLY."
99 Tricia Thompson, February 5, 2020, twitter.com, quoted in Tricia Thompson, "General Mills Proposed Gluten Friendly Line," Gluten Free Watchdog, February 6, 2020. www.glutenfreewatchdog.org
100 Comment in Thompson, "General Milles Proposed."
101 Tricia Thompson, "Gluten Free Watchdog's Updated Position Statement on Cheerios," Gluten Free Watchdog, March 8, 2022, www.glutenfreewatchdog.org.
102 Tricia Thompson, "Gluten-Free Watchdog Cannot Recommend Any Brand of Gluten-Free Oats," Gluten Free Watchdog, April 4, 2023, www.glutenfreewatchdog.org.
103 Jenny Levine Finke, "The Gluten-Free Watchdog Takes Extreme Stance against Gluten-Free Oats," *Good for You* blog, April 5, 2023, www.goodforyouglutenfree.com.
104 "Gluten-Free Oats Remain Complicated as 2023 Comes to a Close," Gluten Free Watchdog, November 2023, www.glutenfreewatchdog.org.
105 Arthur W. Frank, *The Wounded Storyteller: Body, Illness, and Ethics* (Chicago: University of Chicago Press, 1995).

CHAPTER 5. "YOU'RE NOT CRAZY"

1 National Academies of Sciences, Engineering, and Medicine, *Improving Diagnosis in Health Care* (Washington, DC: National Academies Press, 2015), 1.
2 Benjamin Lebwohl and Alberto Rubio-Tapia, "Epidemiology, Presentation, and Diagnosis of Celiac Disease," *Gatroenterology* 160 (2021): 63–75; Daniel A. Leffler, Melinda Dennis, and Benjamin Lebwohl, "Celiac Disease, Chapter 56," in *Yamada's Textbook of Gastroenterology,* seventh edition, ed. Timothy C. Wang et al. (Hoboken, NJ: Wiley, 2022), 1122–36.
3 "An Often-Missed Sign of Celiac Disease," Celiac Disease Foundation, July 2, 2019, https://celiac.org.

4   See Allie B. Cichewicz et al., "Diagnosis and Treatment Patterns in Celiac Disease," *Digestive Diseases and Sciences* 64 (2019): 2095–2106.
5   "Racial Disparities in Celiac Disease Research, Testing, Diagnosis, and Support," Gluten Intolerance Group, June 7, 2021, https://gluten.org.
6   "About," *Michelle's Gluten Free Kitchen*, https://michellesglutenfreekitchen, accessed February 16, 2024.
7   "Welcome to Our Community of Gluten Free Beer Lovers!," Best Gluten Free Beers, https://bestglutenfreebeers.com, accessed February 16, 2024.
8   Denise A. Copelton and Giuseppina Valle, "'You Don't Need a Prescription to Go Gluten-Free': The Scientific Self-Diagnosis of Celiac Disease," *Social Science and Medicine* 69, no. 4 (August 2009): 623–31.
9   Consolato Sergi, Vincenzo Villanacci, and Antonio Carroccio, "Non-Celiac Wheat Sensitivity: Rationality and Irrationality of a Gluten-Free Diet in Individuals Affected with Non-Celiac Disease: A Review," *BMC Gastroenterology* 21, no. 5 (2021); Grazyna Czaja-Bulsa, "Non Coeliac Gluten Sensitivity: A New Disease with Gluten Intolerance," *Clinical Nutrition* 14 (2015): 189–94; Josha Elliott Rubin and Shelia E. Crowe, "In the Clinic: Celiac Disease," *Annals of Internal Medicine*, January 7, 2020; Alessio Fasano, Anna Sapone, Victor Zevallows, and Detief Schuppan, "Nonceliac Gluten Sensitivity," *Gastroenterology* 148 (2015): 1195–1204; Amy C. Brown, "Gluten Sensitivity: Problems of an Emerging Condition Separate from Celiac Disease," *Expert Review of Gastroenterology and Hepatology* 6, no. 1 (2012): 43–55; Maria Raffaella Barbaro et al., "Non-Celiac Gluten Sensitivity in the Context of Functional Gastrointestinal Disorders," *Nutrients* 12, no. 12 (December 4, 2020): 3735.
10 In-person communication, Jimmy Klein and Tom Klein, August 10, 2022, New York, New York.
11 "University of Chicago Celiac Disease Center," University of Chicago, www.uchicago.edu, accessed February 16, 2024.
12 Jerome Groopman, *How Doctors Think* (Boston: Houghton Mifflin, 2007), 12.
13 Groopman, *How Doctors Think*, 6.
14 Debra A. Swoboda, "The Social Construction of Contested Illness Legitimacy: A Grounded Theory Analysis," *Qualitative Research in Psychology* 3 (2008): 233–51.
15 Lisa Sanders, "Hurt All Over," *New York Times Magazine*, November 13, 2011.
16 "Alice Bast's Personal Story," Beyond Celiac, www.beyondceliac.org, accessed February 16, 2024.
17 "About," *Michelle's Gluten Free Kitchen*, https://michellesglutenfreekitchen.wordpress.com, accessed February 16, 2024.
18 Alison St. Sure, "My Story," Surefoodsliving, www.surefoodsliving.com, accessed February 16, 2024.
19 Paula, "A Personal Journey," Celiac Corner, https://celiaccorner.com, accessed February 16, 2024.

20 Susan Wendell, *The Rejected Body: Feminist Philosophical Reflections on Disability* (New York: Routledge, 1996), 122.
21 Erica Dermer, *Celiac and the Beast: A Love Story between a Gluten-Free Girl, Her Genes, and a Broken Digestive Tract* (Celiac and the Beast, 2013).
22 See Suzanne O'Sullivan, *Is It All in Your Head? Stories of Imaginary Illness* (New York: Other Press, 2015).
23 Dermer, *Celiac and the Beast*.
24 Jennifer Esposito, *Jennifer's Way: My Journey with Celiac* (Boston: Da Capo, 2014), 90.
25 Casey Wilson, "Overcoming Motherhood Imposter Syndrome," *New York Times*, April 15, 2020.
26 Ann Campanella, *Celiac Mom: One Family's Gluten-Free Journey after a Daughter's Diagnosis* (Huntersville, NC: Bridge, 2020), 42.
27 Paula, "A Personal Journey."
28 Gluten Dude, "Celiac.com: A Tragic Tale of Good Intentions Gone Awry," *Gluten Dude*, January 17, 2020, https://glutendude.com.
29 See A. R. Lee, R. Wolf, I. Contento, H. Verdell, and P. H. R. Green, "Coeliac Disease: The Association between Quality of Life and Social Support Network Participation," *Journal of Human Nutrition and Dietetics* 29, no. 3 (June 2016): 383–90; Dorothee Köstin, Birte Siem, and Anette Rohmann, "Social Support in Online Peer Groups for Celiac Disease," *European Journal of Health Psychology* 30, no. 3 (2023): 138–43.
30 Quoted in Ryan D. Schroeder and Thomas J. Mowen, "'You Can't Eat WHAT?' Managing the Stigma of Celiac Disease," *Deviant Behavior* 35 (2014): 464.
31 "University of Chicago Celiac Disease Center."
32 David J. Frantz et al., "Cross-Sectional Study of U.S. Interns' Perceptions of Clinical Nutrition Education," *Journal of Parenteral and Enteral Nutrition* 40, no. 4 (2015): 529–35.
33 Stephen Devries, Walter Willett, and Robert O. Bonow, "Nutrition Education in Medical School, Residency Training, and Practice," *JAMA* 3221, no. 14 (April 9, 2019): 1351–52. See also Brian J. Daley et al., "Current Status of Nutrition Training in Graduate Medical Education from a Survey of Residency Program Directors: A Formal Nutrition Education Course Is Necessary," *Journal of Parenteral and Enteral Nutrition* 40, no. 1 (January 2016): 95–99; M Adamski, S. Gibson, M. Leech, and H. Truby, "Are Doctors Nutritionists? What Is the Role of Doctors in Providing Nutrition Advice?," *Nutrition Bulletin* 43 (2018): 147–52.
34 Justin Porter, Cynthia Boyd, M. Reza Skandari, and Neda Laiteerapong, "Revisiting the Time Needed to Provide Adult Primary Care," *Journal of General Internal Medicine* 38, no. 1 (2022): 147–55.
35 Quoted in Devon McPhee, "Primary Care Doctors Would Need More than 24 House in a Day to Provide Recommended Care," *University of Chicago News*, August 11, 2022.

36 All dietitians must be registered; although many nutritionists also are registered, many are not.
37 Alberto Rubio-Tapia, Ivor D. Hill, Carol Semrad, Ciarán P. Kelly, and Benjamin Lebwohl, "American College of Gastroenterology Guidelines Update: Diagnosis and Management of Celiac Disease," *American Journal of Gastroenterology* 118 (2023): 65.
38 Van Waffle, "New Legislation to Extend Medicare Coverage for Dietitian Visits," Celiac Disease Foundation, https://celiac.org, accessed February 17, 2024.
39 Daniel A. Leffler et al., "Factors That Influence Adherence to a Gluten-Free Diet in Adults with Celiac Disease," *Digestive Disease Sciences* 53, no. 6 (June 2008): 1573–81.
40 Si Hari Mahadev et al., "Is Dietitian Use Associated with Celiac Disease Outcomes?," *Nutrients* 5, no. 5 (2013): 1585–94.
41 "Certificate of Training for Gluten Related Disorders from the Academy of Nutrition and Dietetics," Gluten Free Watchdog, August 18, 2020, www.glutenfreewatchdog.org.
42 Van Waffle, "CDF Offers Grants for Dietitians to Complete Gluten-Free Training," Celiac Disease Foundation, https://celiac.org, accessed February 17, 2024.
43 Charles E. Rosenberg, "The Tyranny of Diagnosis: Specific Entities and Individual Experience," *Milbank Quarterly* 80, no. 2 (2002): 240.
44 Leffler, Dennis, and Lebwohl, "Celiac Disease, Chapter 56."
45 Allie B. Cichewicz et al., "Diagnosis and Treatment Patterns in Celiac Disease," *Digestive Disease and Sciences* 64 (2019): 2095–2106.
46 Copelton and Valle, "'You Don't Need a Prescription.'"
47 Steven Epstein, "Measuring Success: Scientific, Institutional, and Cultural Effects of Patient Advocacy," in *Patients as Policy Actors*, ed. Beatrix Hoffman, Nancy Tomes, Rachel Grob, and Mark Schlesinger (New Brunswick, NJ: Rutgers University Press, 2011) 265–66.

CHAPTER 6. BARRIERS TO ADHERENCE

1 World Health Organization, *Adherence to Long-Term Therapies: Evidence for Action* (Geneva: World Health Organization, 2003).
2 Anupam Rej, Luca Elli, and David Surendran Sanders, "Persisting Villous Atrophy and Adherence in Celiac Disease: What Does the Patient Want? What Should a Clinician Advise?," *American Journal of Gastroenterology* 116, no. 5 (May 2021): 946.
3 Dory Sample and Justine Turner, "Improving Gluten Free Diet Adherence by Youth with Celiac Disease," *International Journal of Adolescent Medicine and Health* 33, no. 5 (March 15, 2019); Jacqueline Arnone and Virginia Fitzsimons, "Adolescents with Celiac Disease: A Literature Review of the Impact Developmental Tasks Have on Adherence with a Gluten-Free Diet," *Gastroenterology Nursing* 35, no. 4 (July 2012): 248–54; Gudrun Wagner, "Quality of Life in Adolescents with Treated Coeliac Disease: Influence of Compliance and

Age at Diagnosis," *Journal of Pediatric Gastroenterology and Nutrition* 47, no. 5 (November 2008).

4 Randi L. Wolf et al., "Hypervigilance to a Gluten-Free Diet and Decreased Quality of Life in Teenagers and Adults with Celiac Disease," *Digestive Disease Sciences* 63, no. 6 (June 2018): 1438–48; Jonas F. Ludvigsson et al., "Anxiety after Coeliac Disease Diagnosis Predicts Mucosal Health: A Population-Based Study," *Alimentary Pharmacology & Therapeutics* 48 (2018): 1091–98.

5 See Daniel A. Leffler et al., "Factors That Influence Adherence to a Gluten-Free Diet in Adults with Celiac Disease," *Digestive Disease and Sciences* 53, no. 6 (June 2008): 1573–81; Stefania Paganizza et al., "Is Adherence to a Gluten-Free Diet by Adult Patients with Celiac Disease Influenced by Their Knowledge of the Gluten Content of Foods?," *Gastroenterology Nursing* 42, no. 1 (January/February 2019); N. Barberis, M. C. Quattropani, and F. Cuzzocrea, "Relationship between Motivation, Adherence to Diet, Anxiety Symptoms, Depression Symptoms, and Quality of Life in Individuals with Celiac Disease," *Journal of Psychosomatic Research* 124 (September 2019); Erini Dimidi et al., "Predictors of Adherence to a Gluten-Free Diet in Celiac Disease: Do Knowledge, Attitudes, Experiences, Symptoms, and Quality of Life Play a Role?," *Nutrition* 90 (2021): 1249; Ricardo Fueyo-Díaz et al., "The Effect of Self-Efficacy Expectations in the Adherence to a Gluten-Free Diet in Celiac Disease," *Psychology & Health* 35, no. 6 (2020): 734–49; J. Villafuerte-Galvez et al., "Factors Governing Long-Term Adherence to a Gluten-Free Diet in Adult Patients with Coeliac Disease," *Alimentary Pharmacology & Therapeutics* 42 (2015): 753–60; N. Abu-Janb and M. Jaana, "Facilitators and Barriers to Adherence to Gluten-Free Diet among Adults with Celiac Disease: A Systematic Review," *Journal of Human Nutrition and Dietetics* 33, no. 4 (December 2020): 786–810; Emily J. Kothe et al., "Explaining the Intention-Behaviour Gap in Gluten-Free Diet Adherence: The Moderating Roles of Habit and Perceived Behavioural Control," *Journal of Health Psychology* 20, no. 5 (2015): 580–91; A. J. Dowd et al., "Prediction of Adherence to a Gluten-Free Diet Using Protection Motivation Theory among Adults with Coeliac Disease," *Journal of Human Nutrition and Dietetics* (2015): 391–98; J. A. Silvester et al., "Living Gluten-Free: Adherence, Knowledge, Lifestyle Adaptations, and Feelings towards a Gluten-Free Diet," *Journal of Human Nutrition and Dietetics* 29, no. 3 (June 2016): 374–82; J. A. Silvester et al., "Is It Gluten-Free? Relationship between Self-Reported Gluten-Free Diet Adherence and Knowledge of Gluten Content of Foods," *Nutrition* 32 (2016): 777–83.

6 Nancy Krieger, "Measures of Racism, Sexism, Heterosexism, and Gender Binarism for Health Equity Research from Structural Injustice to Embodied Harm: An Ecosocial Analysis," *Annual Review of Public Health* 41 (2020): 37–62; see Risa J. Lavizzo-Mourey, Richard E. Besser, and David R. Williams, "Understanding and Mitigating Health Inequities: Past, Current, and Future Directions," *New England Journal of Medicine* 384 (May 6, 2021): 1681–84.

7 Sveta Oza et al., "Socioeconomic Risk Factors for Celiac Disease Burden and Symptoms," *Journal of Clinical Gastoenterology* 50, no. 4 (April 2016).
8 Christopher Ma, "Food Insecurity Negatively Impacts Gluten Avoidance and Nutritional Intake in Patients with Celiac," *Journal of Clinical Gastroenterology* 56, no, 10 (November/December 2022): 863–68. See United States Department of Agriculture, Economic Research Service, "Food Security in the U.S.," www.ers.usda.gov, accessed March 31, 2024; Amisha Ahuja, "Comment," *Gastroenterology* 162, no. 7 (June 2022): 2112.
9 Food Research and Action Center, "Hunger and Poverty in America," https://frac.org, accessed February 17, 2024.
10 See, e.g., Gluten Intolerance Group, "5 Ways to Cut Costs on a Gluten-Free Diet," January 7, 2021, https://gluten.org; "Gluten Free on a Budget," Beyond Celiac, www.beyondceliac.org, accessed February 17, 2024.
11 *2022 Annual Report*, Celiac Disease Foundation, https://celiac.org, accessed February 17, 2024.
12 "CDF Leads Effort to Improve Food Security for Women, Infants, and Children with Celiac Disease," Celiac Disease Foundation, February 28, 2022, https://celiac.org.
13 "Gluten-Free Food: A Guide for Food Assistance Organizations," National Celiac Association, June 2020, https://nationalceliac.org.
14 "Gluten Intolerance Group Partners with Cutting Costs for Celiacs," Gluten Intolerance Group, February 16, 2021, https://gluten.org.
15 Margaret Clegg, "Gluten Free Food Assistance in the United States," MI Gluten-Free Gal, November 27, 2023, https://miglutenfreegal.com; Kara Manke, "Gluten-Free Food Banks Bridge Celiac Disease and Hunger," *NPR*, August 7, 2014.
16 Humayun Muhammad et al., "Adherence to a Gluten-Free Diet Is Associated with Receiving Gluten Free Foods on Prescription and Understanding Food Labelling," *Nutrients* 9, no. 7 (July 2017).
17 Emily D. Gutowski et al., "Can Individuals with Celiac Disease Identify Gluten-Free Foods Correctly?," *Clinical Nutrition ESPEN* 36 (April 2020): P82–90.
18 Jeanne Batalova and Elijah Alperin, "Immigrants in the U.S. States with the Fastest-Growing Foreign-Born Populations," Migration Policy Institute, July 10, 2018, www.migrationpolicy.org.
19 Olga Khazan, "Americans Say Immigrants Should Learn English: But U.S. Policy Makes That Hard," *Atlantic*, June 4, 2021.
20 "Hospital Stays Made Safe," Gluten Intolerance Group, April 2022, https://gluten.org.
21 James J. Augustine, "Latest Data Reveal the ED's Role as Hospital Gatekeeper," *ACEP Now*, December 20, 2019.
22 Sarah Curcio, "Celiac Disease and Hospital Care," Celiac.com, July 11, 2019, www.celiac.com.

23 Jennifer Esposito, *Jennifer's Way* (Boston: Da Capo, 2014), 136–37.
24 Jane Anderson, "Does the ADA Cover People with Celiac Disease?," Very Well Health, May 6, 2020, www.verywellhealth.com; Julia Bandini, "'Is It Just Food?': The Social Implications of Celiac Disease as a Disability," *Disability & Society* 30, no. 10 (2015): 1577–81.
25 Isaac Avilucea, "Rider University Settles with Feds over Celiac Disease Complaint, Will Change Dining," *Trentonian*, February 21, 2019.
26 "Celiac Complicates Your College Search," Gluten Free Friends, May 31, 2019, www.gfreefriends.com.
27 "Celiac Complicates Your College Search."
28 "Dear Gluten Dude: My College Won't Keep Me Safe," *Gluten Dude*, September 23, 2015, https://glutendude.com.
29 "Overview of Findings: New England Celiac Organization (NECO) Spring 2016 College Survey," National Celiac Association, August 2016, www.nationalceliac.org.
30 Emily K. Abel, *Elder Care in Crisis: How the Social Safety Net Fails Families* (New York: New York University Press, 2022).
31 Curtiss Ann Matlock, "Nursing Home Care: The Great Challenge for the Celiac," *Journal of Gluten Sensitivity* 15, no. 1 (Winter 2016), www.celiac.com.
32 Matlock, "Nursing Home Care."
33 Abel, *Elder Care in Crisis*, 102.
34 "What Is the Prison Industrial Complex?," Tufts University Prison Divestment, https://sites.tufts.edu, accessed February 17, 2024.
35 Leslie Soble, Kathryn Stroud, and Marika Weinstein, *Eating behind Bars: Ending the Hidden Punishment of Food in Prison*, Impact/Justice, 2020, https://impactjustice.org.
36 "Do Prisons Have Gluten-Free Food?," Gathered Table, June 16, 2022, www.gatheredtable.com.
37 Peter Inserra, "I Told Prison Guards I Have Celiac Disease: They Fed Me Gluten Anyway," *Buzzfeed News*, May 17, 2019, www.buzzfeednews.com.
38 Gene Johnson, "Man Sues Washington Jail over Lack of Gluten-Free Food," *Spokesman-Review*, November 16, 2020; Picciano v. Clark County, WD Washington (1.4.20), 3:20-cv-06106-DGE.

CHAPTER 7. GLUTENED!

1 For summaries of those studies, see Amy Ratner, "Five Years after Diagnosis, More Than Half of Those with Celiac Disease Still Have Symptoms," Beyond Celiac, August 4, 2022, www.beyondceliac.org.
2 Herbert Wieser, Angela Ruiz-Carnicer, Verónica Segura, Isabel Comino, and Carolina Sousa, "Challenges of Monitoring the Gluten-Free Adherence in the Management and Follow-Up of Patients with Celiac Disease," *Nutrients* 13 (2021): 2271.

3   Selvi Rajagopal, "Gluten-Free Diet: Is It Right for Me?," Johns Hopkins Medicine, www.hopkinsmedicine.org, accessed February 17, 2024.
4   A. Rubio-Tapia et al., "American College of Gastroenterology Guidelines Update: Diagnosis and Management of Celiac Disease," *Journal of Gastroenterology* 118 (2023): 65–66; see also F. Fernández-Beñares et al., "Persistent Villous Atrophy in De Novo Adult Patients with Celiac Disease and Strict Control of Gluten-Free Diet Adherence," *American Journal of Gastroenterology* 116 (2021): 1036–43; Alberto Rubio-Tapia et al., "Mucosal Recovery and Mortality in Adults with Celiac Disease after Treatment with a Gluten-Free Diet," *American Journal of Gastroenterology* 105, no. 6 (2010): 1412–20; Peter Haere et al., "Long-Term Mucosal Recovery and Healing in Celiac Disease Is the Rule—Not the Exception," *Scandinavian Journal of Gastroenterology* 51, no. 2 (December 2016): 1439–46; B. Lebwohl et al., "Mucosal Healing and Mortality in Coeliac Disease," *Alimentary Pharmacology & Therapeutics* 37, no. 3 (February 2013): 332–39; Anupam Rej, Luca Elli, and David Surendran Sanders, "Persisting Villous Atrophy and Adherence in Celiac Disease: What Does the Patient Want? What Should a Clinician Advise?," *American Journal of Gastroenterology* 116, no. 5 (May 2021): 946–48.
5   Jocelyn A. Silvester et al., "Most Patients with Celiac Disease on Gluten-Free Diets Consume Measurable Amounts of Gluten," *Gastroenterology* 158 (2020): 1497–99; Juan Pablo Stefano, "Real-World Gluten Exposure in Patients with Celiac Disease on Gluten-Free Diets, Determined from Gliadin Immunogenic Peptides in Urine and Fecal Samples," *Clinical Gastroenterology and Hepatology* 19 (2021): 484–91.
6   Emily Hund, *The Influencer Industry: The Quest for Authenticity on Social Media* (Princeton, NJ: Princeton University Press, 2023).
7   Demetris Vrontis, Anna Makrides, Michael Christofi, and Alkis Thrassou, "Social Media Influencer Marketing: A Systemic Review, Integrative Framework, and Future Research Agenda," *International Journal of Consumer Studies* 45 (2021): 617–44.
8   Vrontis, Makrides, Christofi, and Thrassou, "Social Media Influencer Marketing," 618.
9   J. Kearney Byrne and C. Mac Evilly, "The Role of Influencer Marketing and Social Influencers in Public Health," *Proceedings of the Nutrition Society* 76, issue OCE3: Irish Section Meeting (June 2017); see also "Health Influencers on Social Media: A Threat to Public Health?," Global Health Institute, October 21, 2022, https://globalhealth.georgetown.edu.
10 See Raffael Heiss and Leonie Rudolph, "Patients as Health Influencers: Motivations and Consequences of Following Cancer Patients on Instagram," *Behaviour & Information Technology* 42, no. 6 (2022): 806–15.
11 "Top 1,249 Gluten Free Influencers," Collabstr, https://collabstr.com, accessed February 17, 2024.
12 "Our Mission," Positive Psychology Center, https://ppc.sas.upenn.edu, accessed January 24, 2019.

13 T. Max, "Happiness 101," *New York Times Magazine*, January 7, 2007.
14 David Shimer, "Yale's Most Popular Class Ever: Happiness," *New York Times*, January 26, 2018.
15 Daniel Horowitz, *Happier: The History of a Cultural Movement That Aspired to Transform America* (New York: Oxford University Press, 2018), 5. See also Sara Ahmed, *The Promise of Happiness* (Durham, NC: Duke University Press, 2009); Barbara Ehrenreich, *Bright-Sided: How Positive Thinking Is Undermining America* (New York: Henry Holt, 2009).
16 Erin Smith, "About Me," Gluten Free Globetrotter, https://glutenfreeglobetrotter.com, accessed February 17, 2024.
17 Alison St. Sure, "Speaking & Consulting Services," Sure Foods Living, https://surefoodsliving.com, accessed February 17, 2024.
18 Gluten-Free Optimist: A Positive Slice of Gluten-Free Life, http://glutenfreeoptimist.blogspot.com, accessed February 17, 2024.
19 "My Story," I'm a Celiac, https://www.imaceliac.com, accessed February 17, 2024.
20 "I Like Beer That Doesn't Make Me Sick," Best Gluten Free Beers, https://bestglutenfreebeers.com, accessed February 17, 2024.
21 Alison St. Sure, "My Story," Sure Foods Living, https://surefoodsliving.com, accessed February 17, 2024.
22 Kelly Courson, "About," *Celiac Chicks*, www.celiacchicks.com, accessed May 3, 2021.
23 Smith, "About Me."
24 "My Celiac Diagnosis Story," The Nomadic Fitzpatricks, February 13, 2020, www.thenomadicfitzpatricks.com.
25 Paula Gardner, "A Personal Journey," Celiac Corner, https://celiaccorner.com, accessed February 17, 2024.
26 "About Jennifer," Gluten Free Marcks the Spot, glutenfreemarcksthespot.com, accessed February 17, 2024.
27 Smith, "About Me."
28 See Michel Tuan Pham, Maggie Geuens, and Patrick De Pelsmacker, "The Influence of Ad-Evoked Feelings on Brand Evaluations: Empirical Generalizations from Consumer Responses to More Than 1000 TV Commercials," *International Journal of Research in Marketing* 30, no. 4 (December 2013): 383–94.
29 Jennifer Levine Finke, "Gluten-Free Ravioli Options," Good for You Gluten Free, March 28, 2023, www.goodforyouglutenfree.com.
30 Julie Rosenthal, "About," Goodie Goodie Gluten Free, https://goodiegoodieglutenfree.com, accessed February 17, 2024.
31 Julie Rosenthal, "Health Coaching," Goodie Goodie Gluten Free, https://goodiegoodieglutenfree.com, accessed February 17, 2024.
32 Karina Allrich, "Gluten Free Goddess Tees," Cafepress, www.cafepress.com, accessed February 17, 2024.
33 Quoted in Gluten Dude, "Celiac Disease: Assumptions vs. Reality," *Gluten Dude*, June 25, 2012, https://glutendude.com.

34 Wieser, Ruiz-Carnicer, Segura, Comino, and Sousa, "Challenges of Monitoring the Gluten-Free Diet Adherence."
35 Emily D. Gutowski et al., "Can Individuals with Celiac Disease Identify Gluten-Free Foods Correctly?," *Clinical Nutrition ESPN* 36 (April 2020): 82–90.
36 "Frito-Lay Announces Gluten-Free Certification, Labeling," *Packaging Digest*, March 11, 2015, www.packagingdigest.com.
37 "Note from Alice about Domino's Gluten Free Crust," Beyond Celiac, May 10, 2012, www.beyondceliac.org.
38 Ian Young and Abhinand Thaivalappil, "A Systematic Review and Meta-regression of the Knowledge, Practices, and Training of Restaurant and Food Service Personnel toward Food Allergies and Celiac Disease," *PLoS One* 13, no. 9 (2018): e203496.
39 Benjamin A. Lerner et al., "Detection of Gluten in Gluten-Free Labeled Restaurant Food: Analysis of Crowd-Sourced Data," *American Journal of Gastroenterology* 114, no. 5 (May 2019): 792–97.
40 "Gluten-Free Is Our Drug," *Gluten Dude*, May 27, 2012, https://glutendude.com.

CHAPTER 8. "AN ALIEN IN A STRANGE WORLD"

1 See Richard M. Lee and Steven B. Robbins, "Measuring Belongingness: The Social Connectedness and the Social Assurance Scales," *Journal of Counseling Psychology* 42, no. 2 (1995): 232; Grace Wade, "Frequently Seeing Friends and Family May Cut the Risk of Early Death," *New Scientist*, November 10, 2023; Keith J. Williams and Renee V. Galliher, "Predicting Depression and Self-Esteem from Social Connectedness, Support, and Competence," *Journal of Social and Clinical Psychology* 25, no. 8 (2006): 855–74.
2 Among the many publications that explore the impact of celiac disease on social lives are Ryan D. Schroeder and Thomas J. Mowen, "You Can't Eat WHAT? Managing the Stigma of Celiac Disease," *Deviant Behavior* 35, no.6 (2014): 456–74; A. R. Lee, D. L. Ng, B. Diamond, E. J. Ciaccio, and P. H. R. Green, "Living with Coeliac Disease: Survey Results from the USA," *Journal of Human Nutrition and Dietetics* 25 (2012): 233–38; C. Rose and R. Howard, "Living with Coeliac Disease: A Grounded Theory Study," *Journal of Human Nutrition and Dietetics* 27 (2014): 30–40; Cecilia Olsson et al., "Food That Makes You Different: The Stigma Experienced by Adolescents with Celiac Disease," *Qualitative Health Research* 19, no. 7 (July 2009): 976–84. For a publication that focuses on the impact of celiac disease on work, see Soran R. Bozorg et al., "Work Loss in Patients with Celiac Disease: A Population-Based Longitudinal Study," *Clinical Gastroenterology and Hepatology* 20 (2022): 1068–76.
3 Daniel A. Leffler et al., "Factors That Influence Adherence to a Gluten-Free Diet in Adults with Celiac Disease," *Digestive Disease and Sciences* 53, no. 6 (June 2008): 1573–81.

4. Indeed, sufferers themselves are often unaware of the condition before their diagnosis. "In the past week I've learned that I actually have Celiac Disease," one forum participant wrote. "I'm almost embarrassed to admit that my first reaction was shock to learn that Celiac Disease is a real thing" (June 1, 2016). Another recalled, "I'd heard of celiac disease but was under the impression it was a 'quack disease.' Those words came back to haunt me. I started spending my sleepless nights trying to figure out what in the world was wrong with me, and I found myself on a celiac forum reading about the symptoms of the disease. I had every single symptom but one" (April 6, 2009).
5. "The Mystery of Celiac Disease: The Need for Greater Awareness and Accelerating the Quest for a Cure," Beyond Celiac, May 2022, www.beyondceliac.org.
6. "Mystery of Celiac Disease."
7. Jennifer Esposito, *Jennifer's Way* (Boston: DaCapo, 2014), 133.
8. Even people with gluten intolerance can be blamed for their preoccupation with food. One woman complained to the advice columnist in the *Guardian* about a friend "who has a gluten intolerance and talks about it at length daily. I want her to express her needs, but she doesn't seem to realize that . . . she comes across as high-maintenance and boring." The columnist replied, "To a certain extent the temptation to over-discuss our illnesses is a way to counteract the fact that illness is, necessarily, frustratingly lonely. . . . It's possible your friend has really suffered as a result of this intolerance. Things like Crohn's disease, celiac disease, and many others can land you in pretty serious physical distress." "My Friend's Fixation on Her Gluten Intolerance Puts People Off: Should I Let Her Know?" *Guardian*, September 8, 2023.
9. "Dear Gluten Dude: My Family Members Call Celiac a Fad Disease. Oh . . . and They're Doctors," Gluten Dude, September 13, 2013, https://glutendude.com.
10. A Columbia University study published in 2012 reported that 25 percent of women and 28 percent of men diagnosed within the past two to five years chose not to dine out at all (Lee, Ng, Diamond, Ciaccio, and Green, "Living with Coeliac Disease").
11. See Catharine Rose and Ruth Howard, "Living with Coeliac Disease: A Grounded Theory Study," *Journal of Human Nutrition and Dietetics* 27, no. 1 (February 2014): 30–40.
12. Ellen Samuels, "Passing," in *Keywords for Disability Studies*, ed. Rachel Adams, Benjamin Reiss, and David Serlin (New York: New York University Press, 2015), 135.
13. John R. Porter et al., "Filtered Out: Disability Disclosure Practices on Online Dating Communities," *Proceedings of the ACM: Human Computer Interaction* 1 (November 2017); Fortesa Latifi, "'People Think I'm a Project': The Unique Challenges of Dating with Chronic Illness," *New York Times*, December 28, 2022.
14. Jessica Levbovits et al., "Impact of Celiac Disease on Dating," *Digestive Diseases and Sciences* 67 (2022): 5158–67, https://doi.org/10.1007/s10620-022-07548-y.

15 Esposito, *Jennifer's Way*, 245.
16 Quoted in Schroeder and Mowen, "Managing the Stigma," 469.
17 Quoted in Schroeder and Mowen, "Managing the Stigma," 466.
18 Grayson Seidel, Halle Kotchman, Erin Milner, and Kevin J. O'Donovan, "The Underlying Effects of Celiac Implications on Deployment in the United States Army," *Military Medicine* 187 (March/April 2022): e322.
19 Lee and Robbins, "Measuring Belongingness," 232.
20 See Bozorg et al., "Work Loss."

CONCLUSION

1 Ronald M. Andersen and Pamela Davidson, "Measuring Access and Trends," in *Changing the U.S. Health Care System: Key Issues in Health Services, Policy, and Management*, ed. Ronald M. Andersen, Thomas H. Rice, and Gerald F. Kominski (San Francisco: Jossey-Bass, 1996), 13.
2 Andersen and Davidson, "Measuring Access and Trends," 25.
3 Andersen and Davidson, "Measuring Access and Trends," 25.
4 Margot L. Herman et al., "Patients with Celiac Disease Are Not Followed Up Adequately," *Clinical Gastroenterology and Hepatology* 10 (2012): 893–99.
5 See Steven Epstein, *Impure Science: AIDS, Activism, and the Politics of Knowledge* (Berkeley: University of California Press, 1996).
6 "Food Insecurity," U.S. Department of Health and Human Services: Healthy People 2030, https://health.gov, accessed February 17, 2024.
7 Christopher Ma, "Food Insecurity Negatively Impacts Gluten Avoidance and Nutritional Intake in Patients with Celiac," *Journal of Clinical Gastroenterology* 56, no. 10 (November 2021): 863–68.
8 Bess Williamson, "Access," in *Keywords for Disability Studies*, ed. Rachel Adams, Benjamin Reiss, and David Serlin (New York: New York University Press, 2015), 14–16.
9 Abigail Carroll, *Three Squares: The Invention of the American Meal* (New York: Basic, 2014), 204–5.
10 "Drugs for Celiac Disease May Be on the Horizon," Columbia University Irving Medical Center, May 12, 2022, www.cuimc.columbia.edu.
11 "9 Meters Discontinues Phase 3 Clinical Trial for Potential Celiac Disease Drug Larazotide," Celiac Disease Foundation, June 21, 2022, www.celiac.org. Phase 1 trials focus on safety and side effects. Phase 2 trials determine effectiveness. Phase 3 trials are much larger than the first two; they confirm effectiveness, assess side effects, and compare the drug with existing treatments.
12 Andrew Jacobs, "The Long, Long Wait for a Diabetes Cure," *New York Times*, August 9, 2022.
13 Thomas Insel, "What American Mental-Health Care Is Missing: Scientific Research Alone Cannot Address the Challenges That Americans with Mental Illness Face," *Atlantic*, February 13, 2022.

14. Peter J. Whitehouse with Daniel George, *The Myth of Alzheimer's* (New York: St. Martin's Griffin, 2008); Jason Karlawish, *The Problem of Alzheimer's: How Science, Culture, and Politics Turned a Rare Disease into a Crisis and What We Can Do about It* (New York: St. Martin's, 2021); see Nathan Price and Leroy Hood, "New Alzheimer's Drugs Are Costly and Controversial: Are We Going about It All Wrong?," *Los Angeles Times*, June 11, 2023.
15. Allan M. Brandt, *No Magic Bullet: A Social History of Venereal Disease in the United States since 1880* (New York: Oxford University Press, 1987).
16. Erica Charters, "When Will Covid Really Be Over? Three Things That Will Mark the End of the Pandemic," *Guardian*, July 28, 2022.
17. "Cochlear Implants Pros and Cons: What You Need to Know," The Hearing Solution, February 25, 2019, www.thehearingsolution.com.
18. Chris Feudtner, *Bittersweet: Diabetes, Insulin, and the Transformation of Illness* (Chapel Hill: University of North Carolina Press, 2003), 202.
19. "Hard Truths about Organ Transplants: The Often Harrowing Aftermath," *New York Times*, April 29, 2023.
20. Gina Kolata, "Sickle Cell Cure Brings Mix of Anxiety and Hope," *New York Times*, January 17, 2023.
21. Emily K. Abel and Saskia K. Subramanian, *After the Cure: The Untold Stories of Breast Cancer Survivors* (New York: New York University Press, 2008).

INDEX

Academy of Nutrition and Dietetics, 110
access, 167
access, for people with celiac: disabilities and, 167; to gluten-free food, 47, 168; to health care, 167, 168
ADA. *See* American Diabetes Association; Americans with Disabilities Act
adherence, to medical advice, 113. *See also* gluten-free diet adherence
allergy, 52; celiac as not, 37. *See also* food allergies
Allrich, Karina, 130
AMA. *See* American Medical Association
American Celiac Task Force, 55–56, 75
American College of Gastroenterology, 108, 167
American Diabetes Association (ADA), 70
American Gastroenterological Association, 4; Section on the Diseases of Children, 15
American Journal of Nursing, 22, 25
American Medical Association (AMA), 5
American Pediatric Society, 16, 19
Americans: ignorance of celiac by, 145–49, 169; time spent cooking by, 49, 50; underestimation of celiac by, 145–49
Americans with Disabilities Act (ADA), 118, 123, 124, 165
anaphylactic shock, 53
Andersen, Ronald M., 167
anemia, 98
assisted living facilities, 122, 168

athletes, gluten-free diet and, 38–39, 40–41
awareness of celiac, 12–13; public and medical lack of, 30; social media and, 30

babies: with celiac, 23, 24–25; diarrhea and, 17
Babies Hospital of City of New York, 16–17
Badaracco, Suzy, 32
bananas: babies with celiac and, 23, 24–25; celiac diet and, 20–26, 28; children and, 20–25; children with celiac and, 21, 22, 24–25; food industry and, 20; treatment for celiac with, 9, 20–26; United Fruit Company and, 6, 9, 20, 22–25
Bast, Alice, 46, 73, 84, 97
Belasco, Warren J., 33, 78
Beyond Celiac, 59, 71–74, 97, 145, 192n30
Biltekoff, Charlotte, 34
Brandt, Allan M., 173

Canadian Celiac Association, 88
carbohydrates: celiac and, 21; celiac diet and, 26; intolerance, 19
Carroll, Abigail, 170
CDF. *See* Celiac Disease Foundation
celebrities, gluten-free diet and, 38, 46
celiac: concerns, 103–7; cure, 8; data on, 11–12; difficulties in living with, 2, 131–42; genetics, 2; history, 9, 15, 18–19; misleading comments about, 37; overview, 1. *See also specific topics*

209

celiac advocacy organizations, 7, 10, 29; Cheerios and, 87; corporate funding of, 70, 74–78, 171; corporate sponsorship of, 74–78, 88–89; FALCPA and, 55–58, 75, 171; food industry and, 49, 91–92; gluten-free food industry and, 75–78, 192n30; gluten-free food labeling and, 59, 65–68, 75, 171; gluten-free standards and, 65, 171; major, 70–72; pharmaceutical industry and, 72–75, 171

celiac advocates, 7, 29, 30; CDF and, 89; Cheerios and, 85–87; definition of gluten free and, 58–59, 68; food labeling and, 10, 52, 55–61, 65–68, 171; GM and, 85–87, 89–91

Celiac Chicks, 129

celiac.com, 12, 93, 100, 102–6, 116, 121, 131–65

celiac community, 91

celiac diagnosis, 2, 3; bone loss, 99; celiac influencers, 125, 127, 129; celiac symptoms and, 95–102, 111, 167; difficulty in obtaining, 95–98, 111, 167; difficulty in patient receiving, 103–6; disease label, 99, 101; doctor referrals to dieticians after, 108–9; doctors and, 95–101, 105, 107–9, 111, 167; employment and concealment of, 155; errors in, 93; fears of newly diagnosed patients, 143; gluten challenge, 94; lack of doctor advice on gluten-free diet after, 107–8; misdiagnosed, 98–101, 103; parents of children with, 101–2, 105; patients thinking they're crazy without, 100–101; problems with doctors', 95–101, 105, 111; rise in, 33; risks of other disorders and, 105; self diagnosis, 94–95, 98, 111; technology for, 4, 26–27, 93, 94, 111, 112; as underdiagnosed, 10–11, 93–94, 98–99, 167

celiac diet: bananas and, 20–26, 28; carbohydrates and, 26; children and, 20–23; early historical, 15, 19–23; Haas, Sidney, and, 9, 20–26, 28. *See also* gluten-free diet

celiac disease. *See* celiac

Celiac Disease Center, Columbia University, 31, 72, 76, 110, 172

celiac disease centers, 29

Celiac Disease Foundation (CDF), 71, 72, 74, 76, 78, 110, 115, 171; food industry and, 75, 77, 82, 87, 88, 89, 92; GM and, 87–89, 92

celiac influencers, 30; celiac diagnosis and, 125, 127, 129; celiac recovery and, 125, 126, 127–28; exuberance and good cheer of, 129–30, 142; food industry and, 7, 49; gluten-free diet adherence and, 125; gluten-free diet and, 127–28, 130; gluten-free food marketing and, 130; other marketing by, 130–31; positive psychology movement and, 127

celiac management: doctors and, 3, 6, 11, 108, 168; self management, 4, 107, 109, 111, 112

celiac organizations, 11, 29. *See also* celiac advocacy organizations

celiac recovery: celiac influencers and, 125, 126, 127–28; gluten-free diet adherence and, 11, 113; mucosa damage and, 125; recovery narrative, 8

celiacs. *See* people with celiac

Celiac Sprue Association, 59, 71, 75

celiac symptoms, 2; anemia, 98; asymptomatic, 93; celiac diagnosis and, 95–102, 111, 167; as changing over time, 37; of children with celiac, 29; chronic intestinal indigestion, 17, 19; classic, 98; diarrhea as, 27, 29, 161–62; doctors and, 94; employment and, 7, 93, 156–63, 165; fatigue, 156; gastrointestinal, 93, 96, 98, 131–33; after being glutened,

43, 125–26, 131–42, 157, 158; gluten-free diet adherence and persistent, 125; gluten-free diet and, 8, 125; lack of external, 8, 169; stomach aches, 131–32; as varied, 1, 28, 93
Center for Food Safety and Applied Nutrition, FDA, 63, 67
cereal: Chex, 75, 79; GM's Cheerios, 10, 75, 77–92, 194n61; GM's other, 78; health and, 79
cereal manufacturers, 78. *See also* General Mills
Certificate of Training for Gluten-Related Disorders, 110
Charters, Erica, 173
Cheerios: celiac advocates and, 85–87; complaints about, 81–91; GFWD and, 82, 83, 90, 91; gluten-free, 10, 75, 77–92, 194n61; GMO-free, 80–81; recall of contaminated, 85–86; wheat and, 85–86
Chex cereals, 75, 79
children: bananas and, 20–25; celiac and, 20–23; celiac diet and, 20–23; cereal manufacturers and, 78; *Diseases of Infancy and Childhood*, 16; food marketing and, 49, 78; obesity, 78
children with celiac: bananas and, 21, 22, 24–25; celiac symptoms of, 29; gluten-free diet and, 27; parents of, 101–2, 105, 118; public schools and, 118; United Fruit Company and, 24–25
chronic intestinal indigestion, 17, 19
coeliac, 15, 21
colleges and universities: gluten-free diet adherence in, 118–20; positive psychology courses at, 126–27. *See also specific colleges and universities*
Columbia University, Celiac Disease Center, 31, 72, 76, 110, 172
commercialism, medicine and, 4–5
cookbooks, gluten-free food, 38, 42, 48

cooking: Americans' time spent, 49, 50; food industry and, 49–50; gluten-free food, 48–51; time spent on gluten-free food, 50–51
"Coping with Celiac Disease" forum, 12
corporate funding: celiac advocacy organizations and, 70, 74–78, 171; of HAOs, 69–70, 190n1
corporate sponsorship: celiac advocacy organizations and, 74–78, 88–89; gluten-free food marketing and, 77, 78; of HAOs, 70
Courson, Kelly, 128–29

Danyluk, Kim, 128–29
dating, of people with celiac, 153–54
Davis, William, 35, 36–38
Deaver, Debby, 32
Department of Agriculture, US, 5, 62, 115
Department of Health and Human Services, US, 5, 58
Department of Justice, US, 118
depression, 143, 144
diabetes, 70, 109, 173
diagnosis, 110; health care errors in, 93. *See also* celiac diagnosis
diagnostic technology: intestinal biopsy, 26–27, 93, 94; patient self-reports compared to, 4; serological tests, 93; for testing for celiac, 4, 26–27, 93, 94, 111, 112
diarrhea: babies and, 17; as celiac symptom, 27, 29, 161–62; employment of people with celiac and, 161–62
diet: bananas in, 20–23; early 20th century, 22; health and, 33
Dietary Goals for the United States, 33
Dietary Guidelines, 5, 177n9
dieticians, 168, 199n36; deficiencies regarding celiac care by, 109–10; doctor referrals after celiac diagnosis to, 108–9; proposed training on gluten-free diet for, 110. *See also* nutritionists

disabilities: access for people with celiac and, 167; people with, 7–8; social model of, 169
disclosure problems, of people with celiac, 8–9; employment and, 154–57; in social life, 153–54
Diseases of Infancy and Childhood (Holt), 16
Disney, 41, 44
Djokovic, Novak, 39
doctors: celiac appointments with, 156, 167; celiac diagnosis and, 95–101, 105, 107–9, 111, 167; celiac management and, 3, 6, 11, 108, 168; celiac symptoms and, 94; food industry and, 6; gluten-free diet and, 48, 107–8; inability to rely for treatment on, 111; lack of advice on gluten-free diet after celiac diagnosis by, 107–8; late 19th/early 20th century, 15–17; low knowledge of celiac by, 30, 108; medical knowledge of patients and, 67; nutrition and, 16, 108; problems with celiac diagnosis by, 95–101, 105, 111; referrals to dieticians after celiac diagnosis, 108–9. *See also* pediatricians

"Eat!Gluten-Free" app, 76–77
employment, of people with celiac, 143; accommodations in, 157, 159; blue and white-collar workers, 165; celiac diagnosis concealment and, 155; celiac symptoms and, 7, 93, 156–63, 165; childcare work, 160–61; diarrhea and, 161–62; disqualifications for work, 163–64; fear of loss of respect from coworkers, 159; fear of reprisals in, 158–59; gluten-free diet and, 11; lack of support from bosses, 157–59, 169; problems with celiac disclosure in, 154–57; professional and managerial positions, 162–63; travel issues, 155, 157, 158, 161–63; working part-time or quitting, 163; work loss, 165
epidemics, 173
Epstein, Steven, 112
Esposito, Jennifer, 100, 117–18, 146, 153–54
ethnic and religious communities, 164–65
European research, on celiac, 9, 18, 26–29

FAAN. *See* Food Allergy and Anaphylaxis Network
FALCPA. *See* Food Allergen Labeling and Consumer Protection Act
Fallon, Jimmy, 44
family and friends, 145–52, 164–65, 169–70
Fasano, Alessio, 28–29, 46, 55, 59, 181n62
FDA. *See* Food and Drug Administration
Feudtner, Chris, 173
Flexner, Simon, 18
Folayan, Sabaah, 41
food: GMO-free, 80–81; organic, 78; overproduction, 5. *See also* gluten-free food
Food Allergen Labeling and Consumer Protection Act (FALCPA), 10, 54–58, 75, 139, 171
food allergens: food labeling and, 10, 54–58, 75, 139, 171; gluten as, 56
food allergies, 40; activists, 53–54; anaphylactic shock from, 53; celiac and, 52; dangers of, 53; GM and, 79; restaurants and, 43–44. *See also* gluten sensitivity
Food Allergy and Anaphylaxis Network (FAAN), 53, 54, 70, 187n5
Food and Drug Administration (FDA), 3, 10, 173; Center for Food Safety and Applied Nutrition, 63, 67; food industry and, 64, 66, 67, 89, 90; food labeling and, 54, 55, 56, 59–68, 75, 89,

90; gluten-free food and, 58–68, 72, 75, 89, 90
food deserts, 47
food faddism, Golden Age of, 22
food industry: bananas and, 20; CDF, 75, 77, 82, 87, 88, 89, 92; celiac advocacy organizations and, 49, 91–92; celiac influencers and, 7, 49; cooking and, 49–50; definition of gluten free and, 64, 68; Dietary Guidelines and, 5, 177n9; doctors and, 6; FDA and, 64, 66, 67, 89, 90; food labeling and, 54–58, 60, 61, 66, 67, 137; gluten-free food and, 47, 52, 60–61, 64, 66–68, 76–81, 136–37; gluten-free food industry, 9, 75–78, 192n30; HAOs and, 70; medicine and, 5; organic and natural food and, 78; overeating and, 5, 6; people with celiac and, 4, 6–7, 136–37. *See also specific food companies*
food labeling: celiac advocates and, 10, 52, 55–61, 65–68, 171; celiac and, 9–10, 55–61, 135–39; FALCPA, 10, 54–58; FDA and, 54, 55, 56, 59–68, 75, 89, 90; food allergens and, 10, 54–58, 75, 139, 171; food industry and, 54–58, 60, 61, 66, 67, 137; FOPL, 52, 54; gluten friendly, 89–90; GM and, 79; inadequacies of, 54; natural, 78; *New York Times* and, 54, 55; Nutrition Labeling and Education Act, 52. *See also* gluten-free food labeling
food marketing, 48; children and, 49, 78; gluten-free, 49, 77, 78, 130; obesity and, 49, 78
food safety, 62, 63–64
The Food Value of the Banana, 20, 23
FOPL. *See* front-of-packaging labeling
Freidson, Eliot, 4
Frito-Lays chips, 137
front-of-packaging labeling (FOPL), 52, 54

Gardner, Paula, 98, 102, 129
gastroenterologists, 2, 3, 9, 28, 98; American Gastroenterological Association, 4, 15
gastrointestinal celiac symptoms, 93, 96, 98, 131–33
Gee-Herter Disease, 18
Gee, Samuel, 15, 18, 21
Geller, Marilyn, 73, 82, 87
General Mills (GM): CDF and, 87–89, 92; celiac advocates and, 85–87, 89–91; Cheerios, 10, 75, 77–92, 194n61; Chex cereals, 75, 79; criticisms of, 81–91; food allergies and, 79; food labeling and, 79; Gluten Dude and, 81, 82, 84, 86, 89; gluten-free food market and, 47, 78–81, 87–88; gluten-free forum, 81; gluten-free testing by, 79, 82–84, 86–88; gluten friendly food of, 89–90; misleading claims by, 80–90, 194n61; other cereals of, 78; Rice Chex, 79
GFWD. *See* Gluten Free Watchdog
GIG. *See* Gluten Intolerance Group
gluten: as allergen, 56; celiac caused by, 2, 26–27; inability to process, 36; obesity and, 35. *See also specific topics*
gluten avoidance, external: kitchen cleaning, 106–7; topical exposure, 105
gluten challenge, 94
Gluten Dude, 45, 102, 119, 131, 139, 148, 169; GM and, 81, 82, 84, 86, 89
glutened, 43, 125–26, 131–42, 155, 157, 158, 161–62, 170
gluten free, definition of, 58–59, 60, 63, 64, 68
gluten-free diet, 76; accommodation of, 40; athletes and, 38–39, 40–41; celebrities and, 38, 46; celiac influencers and, 125, 127–28, 130; celiac symptoms and, 8, 125; children with celiac and, 27; conditions caused and cured by, 36;

gluten-free diet (*cont.*)
doctors and, 48, 107–8; employment and, 11; extreme measures taken by people with celiac, 146–48; gluten-free food labeling and, 46–47, 116; knowledge by people with celiac of, 109; lack of doctor advice after celiac diagnosis on, 107–8; media and, 38–42; popularity of, 31, 38; publicity of, 39; race and, 41–42; social life and, 11, 30; as time consuming, 46–47, 50; training for dieticians on, 110; as treatment for celiac, 3, 4, 9, 26–28, 39, 46; trivialization and criticism of, 39–45, 169; wealth and, 42

gluten-free diet adherence: assistance for, 115, 124; assisted living facilities and, 122, 168; celiac influencers and, 125; celiac recovery and, 11, 113; celiac symptoms persisting after, 125; in colleges and universities, 118–20; compliance compared to, 10; difficulties in, 10–11, 13, 103–8, 113–24, 133–42, 168; factors in, 113–15, 124, 168, 173; food insecurity and, 115; gluten-free food labeling and, 116, 135–39; hospital admissions and, 116–18; institutions and, 116–24, 168; language difficulties in, 116; medical professionals and, 143; nursing homes and, 120–22, 168; in prisons and jails, 123–24, 168; rates of, 113; ridicule of, 31; studies of, 11, 113; vigilance required in, 4, 106–7, 113, 142

Gluten Free Expo, Sandy, Utah, 32

gluten-free food, 2, 3; access to, 47, 168; availability of, 46; boom in, 32–33, 38; Cheerios as, 10, 75, 77–92, 194n61; cookbooks, 38, 42, 48; cooking, 48–51; costs and benefits, 45–47, 51; as expensive, 31, 47, 113–14, 168; FALCPA and, 56, 57, 58; FDA and, 58–68, 72, 75, 89, 90; flavor, 47; food industry and, 47, 52, 60–61, 64, 66–68, 76–81, 136–37; foods naturally free of gluten, 31, 76; health and, 31, 45–46; meal plans, 77; *New York Times* on, 63; processed food and, 31, 48, 50; recipes, 38, 39; restaurants and, 40, 43–44, 139–42, 170; standards, 64–68, 89, 171; testing of, 71–72, 79, 82–84, 86–88; time spent cooking, 50–51; as unappealing, 47; as unhealthy, 31, 45–46; weight and, 34, 35; wheat-free food and, 57

gluten-free food industry, 9, 75–78, 192n30

gluten-free food labeling, 57–58, 60–64, 79, 82–83, 87–88, 90; celiac advocacy organizations and, 59, 65–68, 75, 171; GFWD and, 65, 67; gluten-free diet adherence and, 116, 135–39; gluten-free diet and, 46–47, 116; inadequacies of, 135–39; restaurants and, 139

gluten-free food market, 9, 31; GM and, 47, 78–81, 87–88; growth of, 32–33, 51

gluten-free food marketing: celiac influencers and, 130; corporate sponsorship and, 77, 78; direct to celiacs, 49

Gluten-Free Globetrotter, 129

Gluten-Free Goddess, 130

gluten free influencers, 126. *See also* celiac influencers

Gluten Free Watchdog (GFWD), 74–75, 171; Cheerios and, 82, 83, 90, 91; gluten-free food labeling and, 65, 67; gluten testing and, 71–72

gluten friendly label, 89–90

gluten intolerance, 206n8

Gluten Intolerance Group (GIG), 70, 75, 115, 116

gluten sensitivity: celiac and, 95; nonceliac, 33, 46

GM. *See* General Mills

GMO-free food, Cheerios, 80–81

Grain Brain (Perlmutter), 35–38

Green, Peter H. R., 31
Groopman, Jerome, 96, 97, 111–12
Guandalini, Stefano, 28

Haas, Merrill, 25, 26, 27
Haas, Sidney V., 9, 20–28
HAOs. *See* health-advocacy organizations
Hawley, Paul, 5
health: cereal and, 79; diet and, 33; gluten-free food and, 31, 45–46; unhealthiness of processed food, 52; US government and, 33–34; weight and, 34, 35
health-advocacy organizations (HAOs), 69–70, 73, 190n1
health care: diagnosis errors, 93; lack of insurance, 94; people with celiac and access to, 167, 168
health disparities research, 113
health problems, from celiac, 1–2
Herter, Christian, 18, 19
Holt, L. Emmett, Jr., 27
Holt, Luther Emmett, 16–20
hospital admissions, gluten-free diet adherence and, 116–18
household members, lack of support from, 144–50, 164
How Doctors Think (Groopman), 96, 97
Howland, John, 19, 20, 21

Insel, Thomas P., 172
Institute of Medicine, 63
institutions: access to gluten-free food in, 168; gluten-free diet adherence and, 116–24, 168. *See also specific institutions*
intestinal biopsy, 26–27, 93, 94
intestinal infantilism, 18–19
isolation and loneliness, 11, 30, 104, 143, 144

Journal of the American Medical Association, 20

Kamen, Paula, 8
Kennedy, Edward M., 54, 55, 56
Kohut, Heinz, 164

Leahy, Patrick, 62–63
Lesley University, 118
Levario, Andrea, 29, 55, 56, 57, 60
Lloyd-Still, John D., 27, 28
Lowey, Nita M., 54, 55, 56
Lubet, Steven, 8

Matlock, Curtiss Ann, 120–21
McGovern, George, 33
media coverage of celiac: gluten-free diet, 38–42; as vanishing between 1969 and 1982, 28
medical professionals: gluten-free diet adherence and, 143. *See also* doctors
medical schools: nutrition education, 108. *See also specific medical schools*
Medicare, 120, 121
medicine: adherence to medical advice, 113; commercialism and, 4–5; food industry and, 5
Monsanto Company, 62
Morse, John Lovett, 23
mucosa damage, 112, 125
Muñoz-Furlong, Anne, 53, 54, 55
Myers, Victor C., 20, 21

National Academies of Sciences, Engineering, and Medicine, 93
National Celiac Association (NCA), 71, 75, 115, 119
National Foundation for Celiac Awareness (NFCA), 71, 81, 84
National Institutes of Health, 29
natural food, 78
Nature Valley, 75
NCA. *See* National Celiac Association
Nestle, Marion, 62, 80–81
New York Academy of Medicine, 21, 25

New York Times, 23, 24, 28, 32, 38, 47, 53; food labeling and, 54, 55; on gluten-free food, 63
NFCA. *See* National Foundation for Celiac Awareness
No Magic Bullet (Brandt), 173
Non-celiac gluten sensitivity, 33, 46, 95. *See also* gluten sensitivity
North, Jennifer, 81
nursing homes, 120–22, 168
nutrition: doctors and, 16, 108; medical school education in, 108; pediatrics and, 16–17; weight gain and, 17
nutritionists, 108, 168, 199n36; ignorance of celiac by, 109. *See also* dieticians
Nutrition Labeling and Education Act (1990), 52, 62

oats, 80, 81, 82, 88, 91
obesity, 34; children and, 78; food marketing and, 49, 78; gluten and, 35; highly processed food and, 5
On Infantilism from Chronic Intestinal Infection (Herter), 18
organic food, 78
overeating, food industry and, 5, 6
overtreatment, 5
overweight, 34, 35

parents, of children with celiac, 101–2, 105, 118
passing, 153, 155, 169
patients: doctors' obligation to, 5; medical knowledge of doctors and, 67
patient self-reports, diagnostic technology compared to, 4
pediatricians, 15–16
pediatrics, nutrition and, 16–17
people with celiac, 33; access to health care for, 167, 168; as activists, 171; ambivalence about asking for help, 169–70; disclosure problems of, 8–9, 153–57; extreme measures in gluten-free diet taken by, 146–48; food industry and, 4, 6–7, 136–37; ideology of personal responsibility and, 170; ignorance of celiac by, 206n4; knowledge of gluten-free diet by, 109; lack of sympathy for, 8, 169; lack of understanding of, 30, 169; pharmaceutical industry and, 7, 72–73; political/social reforms needed to help, 172, 173; in poverty, 168; protests against trivialization of gluten-free diet by, 44–45; self-blame of, 11, 141–42, 170–71; self-management, 4, 107, 109, 111, 112; social media influencers and, 11; subjective knowledge of, 96, 111–12; as undiagnosed and neglected, 29. *See also* employment, of people with celiac; *specific topics*
Perlmutter, David, 35–38
personal responsibility, ideology of, 170
pharmaceutical drugs, treatment for celiac using, 7, 30, 72–73, 91, 171–73, 207n11
pharmaceutical industry: celiac advocacy organizations and, 72–75, 171; HAOs and, 69, 70, 73; people with celiac and, 7, 72–73; research on celiac treatments, 72–73
Podell, David, 97
Positive Psychology Center, University of Pennsylvania, 126–27
positive psychology movement, 126–27, 144
prisons and jails, 123–24, 168
processed food: gluten-free food and, 31, 48, 50; obesity and highly, 5; ultraprocessed, 31, 76; unhealthiness of, 52

Reagan, Ronald, 33–34
recipes, gluten-free food, 38, 39

Rehabilitation Act (1973), 118, 124, 165
research on celiac, 74; European, 9, 18, 26–29; US, 18, 27–29. *See also specific topics*
research on celiac treatment, 26–29; pharmaceutical industry and, 72–73; vaccine or cure, 73–74
restaurants: food allergies and, 43–44; glutened at, 139–42, 170; gluten-free food and, 40, 43–44, 139–42, 170; gluten-free food labeling at, 139
Rice Chex, gluten-free, 79
Rider University, 118–19
Rockefeller Institute for Medical Research, 16, 18
Rockefeller, John D., Jr., 16
Rose, Anton R., 20, 21
Rosenberg, Charles E., 110–11
Rosenthal, Julie, 130
Rose, Sarah F., 7

Sanders, Lisa, 97
schools: public, 118. *See also* colleges and universities; medical schools
Schor, Juliet B., 50
self-control, 34, 36
Seligman, Martin, 126
serological tests, 93
Shapiro, Laura, 49
Shiner, Margot, 26
Smith, Erin, 84–85, 129
social disconnectedness, of people with celiac: avoidance of eating out, 143, 144, 149, 206n10; avoidance of offending those who love to share food, 153; avoidance of social engagements, 143, 144; dating and, 153–54; depression, 143, 144; discussions on celiac.com about, 143–65; due to struggles to blend in, 153; employment and, 154–65; ethnic and religious diets and, 164–65; fear of loss of respect from coworkers, 159; feelings of being an inconvenience and, 151–52, 159, 170; guilt and shame in, 151–52; isolation and loneliness, 11, 30, 104, 143, 144; lack of support from bosses, 157–59, 169; lack of support from household members, 144–50, 164; "passing" in, 153, 155; problems of celiac disclosure in employment, 154–57; problems of celiac disclosure in social life, 153–54; problems with family and friends, 145–52, 164–65, 169–70; quitting work, 163; restaurants and, 149, 157–58, 162, 206n10; travel and, 155, 157, 158, 161–63
social life, of people with celiac, 143; disclosure problems in, 153–54; gluten-free diet and, 11, 30. *See also* social disconnectedness, of people with celiac
social media, awareness of celiac and, 30
social media influencers, 126; people with celiac and, 11. *See also* celiac influencers
stomach aches, 131–32
support groups, celiac, 29–30
The Surgeon General's Call to Action to Prevent and Decrease Overweight and Obesity, 34
surgeon general, US, 33, 34
surgery, unnecessary, 5
Swidey, Neil, 43

Taylor, Michael R., 61–63, 64
testing: for celiac, 4, 26–27, 93, 94, 111, 112; GFWD and gluten, 71–72; of gluten-free food, 71–72, 79, 82–84, 86–88; serological tests, 93; unnecessary tests, 5–6
thinness, 34–35
Thompson, Tricia, 65–67, 71, 74–75, 82–86, 90, 91

travel, 155, 157, 158, 161–63
treatment for celiac: bananas as, 9, 20–26; gluten-free diet as, 3, 4, 9, 26–28, 39, 46; inability to rely on doctors for, 111; pharmaceutical drugs as, 7, 30, 72–73, 91, 171–73, 207n11; research on, 26–29, 72–74

UFC. *See* United Fruit Company
ultraprocessed food, 31, 76
United Fruit Company (UFC): bananas and, 6, 9, 20, 22–25; celiac and, 24–25, 28; Haas and, 23–24
United States (US): celiac as neglected in, 29; *Dietary Goals for the United States*, 33; health and, 33–34; medical certification of celiac in, 29; research on celiac, 18, 27–29; resurgence of interest in celiac in 1990s, 28
University of Chicago Celiac Disease Center, 28, 95, 107
University of Chicago Medical School, 28
University of Maryland: Center for Celiac Research, 28, 55, 181n62; Medical School, 28
US. *See* United States

"The Value of the Banana in the Treatment of Celiac Disease" (Haas), 20

weight: gluten-free food and, 34, 35; health and, 34, 35; nutrition and, 17; overweight, 34, 35; wheat and, 35
Wendell, Susan, 99
wheat: Cheerios and, 85–86; gluten-free food and wheat-free food, 57; weight and, 35
Wheat Belly (Davis), 35, 36–38
women: housework and, 50; thinness and, 34–35
World Health Organization, 10, 48
Wyden, Ron, 62–63

ABOUT THE AUTHOR

EMILY K. ABEL is Professor Emerita at the Fielding School of Public Health, University of California, Los Angeles. She is the author of many books, including *Limited Choices: Mable Jones, a Black Children's Nurse in a Northern White Household*, coauthored with Margaret K. Nelson, and *Elder Care in Crisis: How the Social Safety Net Fails Families* (New York University Press).

www.ingramcontent.com/pod-product-compliance
Lightning Source LLC
Chambersburg PA
CBHW020406080526
44584CB00014B/1203